Analysis File of Drug-Induced Lung Injury

Akihiko Gemma

Analysis File of Drug-Induced Lung Injury

Expert Opinion for Analysis of Big Data

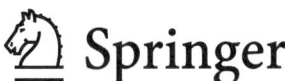

Akihiko Gemma
Department of Pulmonary Medicine and Oncology
Graduate School of Medicine, Nippon Medical School
Bunkyo-ku, Tokyo, Japan

ISBN 978-981-97-3448-1   ISBN 978-981-97-3446-7   (eBook)
https://doi.org/10.1007/978-981-97-3446-7

Translation from the Japanese language edition: "Yakuzaisei Hai Shougai Bunseki Fairu" by Akihiko Gemma, © Nankodo Co., Ltd. 2021. Published by Nankodo Co., Ltd. All Rights Reserved.

© The Editor(s) (if applicable) and The Author(s), under exclusive license to Springer Nature Singapore Pte Ltd. 2024
This work is subject to copyright. All rights are solely and exclusively licensed by the Publisher, whether the whole or part of the material is concerned, specifically the rights of reprinting, reuse of illustrations, recitation, broadcasting, reproduction on microfilms or in any other physical way, and transmission or information storage and retrieval, electronic adaptation, computer software, or by similar or dissimilar methodology now known or hereafter developed.
The use of general descriptive names, registered names, trademarks, service marks, etc. in this publication does not imply, even in the absence of a specific statement, that such names are exempt from the relevant protective laws and regulations and therefore free for general use.
The publisher, the authors and the editors are safe to assume that the advice and information in this book are believed to be true and accurate at the date of publication. Neither the publisher nor the authors or the editors give a warranty, expressed or implied, with respect to the material contained herein or for any errors or omissions that may have been made. The publisher remains neutral with regard to jurisdictional claims in published maps and institutional affiliations.

This Springer imprint is published by the registered company Springer Nature Singapore Pte Ltd.
The registered company address is: 152 Beach Road, #21-01/04 Gateway East, Singapore 189721, Singapore

If disposing of this product, please recycle the paper.

Preface

Overview: Experience of Drug-Induced Lung Injury Exploratory Committee

Drug-induced lung injury is a pathologic condition often seen during current common medical care using many drugs. Presently, drugs are considered a significant factor for inducing pulmonary lesions presenting diffuse haziness.

Recently, there is a worldwide race to develop molecular target treatment drugs and the globalization of the clinical developmental process has advanced. In the cancer treatment field, the number of clinical trial studies with Japanese subjects has decreased. However, variations between races in the occurrence of drug-induced lung injury have been reported. Of note, it is reported that Japanese people are more susceptible to diffuse alveolar damage (DAD), leading to poor prognosis. Although drug-induced lung injury, a harmful event with a low frequency, is recognized as having different rates of occurrence between races, the disorder remains insufficiently analyzed. Despite this situation, the drugs' approvals and use have become inevitable.

However, in such situation in Japan, unprecedented surveys in comparison with other countries, that is, post-marketing all-case surveys limited to large-scale facilities have been performed. The surveys permit the collection of relatively accurate and sufficient information about drug-induced lung injuries and provide some clarity on the situation. The surveys and analyses have produced an accurate frequency of drug-induced lung injuries, risk factors, and pathologic conditions. The accumulated information has become important knowledge for appropriate uses of drugs. As for evidence for harmful events, it is considered appropriate to analyze big data whose case-selection bias is low because the case selection approximates that in the clinical setting.

In this book, I have outlined my understanding and point of view through the experiences of an exploratory committee of big-data analyses of drug-induced lung injuries. Chapter 1 is a summary of the pathologic conditions and factors of drug-induced lung injuries, idea of the monitoring, and cautions in looking at the evidence. In Chapter 2, the results of post-marketing all-case surveys, characteristic pathologic conditions revealed by the surveys, cautions at administration, notable topics, and inside stories of my experiences are put together for individual drugs. Please note that in introducing important topics and cautions, the papers and materials of information disclosure from the companies may be presented when necessary, because it is rare to be presented as a final paper and there is some important information shown with partial disclosure of information from companies. In addition, the statistics are not up-to-date because they show the realistic sense of drug-induced lung injury management, as they are at the time of management.

Accordingly, this book does not outline the basic knowledge of ordinary drug-induced lung injuries but instead contains a lot of content which is not in other books such as the guidelines edited by the academic society and instructional texts. The goal of this book is to be used as a reference at the management level of drug-induced lung injury as well as in clinical use for treatment of the respiratory organs and cancers. I hope that this book will become useful for unique experiences and difficult situations.

Bunkyo-ku, Tokyo, Japan Akihiko Gemma
April 2023

Contents

Part I Understanding Drug-Induced Lung Injuries

1 Understanding Drug-Induced Lung Injuries.................... 3
   1.1 Pathologic Conditions of Drug-Induced Lung Injuries
       and Factors Inferred from Big Data......................... 3
       1.1.1 Mechanism of Onset 3
       1.1.2 Pathologic Conditions 3
       1.1.3 Treatments 4
       1.1.4 Factors Inferred from Big Data 4
   1.2 Practice of the Monitoring................................. 7
       1.2.1 EGFR Tyrosine Kinase Inhibitors (EGFR-TKI) 8
       1.2.2 mTOR inhibitors and Immune Checkpoint Inhibitors..... 8
       1.2.3 Cases with Risk Factors and Prognosis Factors.......... 9
   1.3 Cautions in Interpreting the Big Data Evidence 9
       1.3.1 Consideration of the Lung Damage................... 9
       1.3.2 Specificity of the First-in-Class Drug 10
       1.3.3 Pulmonary Thromboembolism as Differential Diagnoses.. 11
       1.3.4 Conforming Parameters........................... 11
   References.. 11

Part II Actual Practice in Drug-Induced Lung Injuries of Each Drug

**2 EGFR Inhibitors (Gefitinib, Erlotinib, Afatinib,
and Osimertinib)**... 15
   2.1 Gefitinib (Iressa) 15
       2.1.1 An in-Cohort Case-Controlled Study in Patients with
            Lung Cancer as Subjects 15
       2.1.2 Findings from the Surveys......................... 18
   2.2 Erlotinib (Tarceva)...................................... 22
       2.2.1 Post-Marketing all-Case Survey in Patients with
            Non-small Cell Lung Cancer....................... 22

		2.2.2	Findings from the Survey.	24
		2.2.3	Specific Survey of Use Achievement in Patients with Pancreatic Cancer (All-Case Survey)	24
		2.2.4	Findings from the Survey.	25
		2.2.5	Findings from the Survey.	27
	2.3	Afatinib (Gilotrif).		28
		2.3.1	Post-Marketing All-Case Survey in Subjects with Non-small Cell Lung Cancer.	28
		2.3.2	Findings from the Survey.	29
	2.4	Osimertinib (Tagrisso).		29
		2.4.1	Post-Marketing All-Case Survey in Subjects with Non-small Cell Lung Cancer.	31
		2.4.2	Findings from the Survey.	31
	2.5	Vandetanib (Caprelsa).		34
	References.			34
3	**Anti-EGFR Antibodies (Cetuximab, Panitumumab, and Necitumumab).**			**37**
	3.1	Cetuximab (Erbitux).		37
		3.1.1	Post-Marketing All-Case Survey in Colon and Rectal Cancers.	37
		3.1.2	Findings from the Survey.	39
	3.2	Panitumumab (Vectibix).		42
		3.2.1	Post-Marketing All-Case Survey in Patients with Colon and Rectal Cancers.	42
		3.2.2	Findings from the Survey.	42
	3.3	Necitumumab (Portrazza).		45
		3.3.1	Post-Marketing Survey in Patients with Squamous Cell Lung Cancer.	45
	References.			45
4	**mTOR Inhibitors (Temsirolimus and Everolimus).**			**47**
	4.1	Temsirolimus (Torisel).		47
	4.2	Everolimus (Afinitor).		47
		4.2.1	Post-Marketing All-Case Survey in Patients with Renal Cell Cancer.	48
		4.2.2	Findings from the Surveys.	48
	References.			57
5	**Proteasome Inhibitor (Bortezomib).**			**59**
	5.1	Bortezomib (Velcade).		59
		5.1.1	Topic.	59
		5.1.2	Findings from the Survey.	60
	References.			62

6	**Immune Checkpoint Inhibitors (Nivolumab, Pembrolizumab, Atezolizumab, and Durvalumab)**................................		63
	6.1	Nivolumab (Opdivo)	63
		6.1.1 All-Case Survey in Subjects with Non-small Cell Lung Cancer..................................	63
		6.1.2 Findings from the Surveys........................	65
	6.2	Pembrolizumab (Keytruda)	69
		6.2.1 Usage-Achievement Surveys in Subjects with Malignant Melanoma and Non-small Cell Lung Cancer...	69
		6.2.2 Findings from the Surveys........................	72
	6.3	Atezolizumab (Tecentriq)	72
		6.3.1 Early Post-Marketing Surveys in Subjects with Non-small Cell Lung Cancer......................	72
	6.4	Durvalumab (Imfinzi)	72
		6.4.1 Topic	73
	References..		74
7	**Neoangiogenesis Inhibitors (Sunitinib, Sorafenib, and Bevacizumab)**		75
	7.1	Sunitinib (Sutent)...................................	75
		7.1.1 Post-Marketing All-Case Survey in Subjects with Renal Cell Cancer	75
		7.1.2 Findings from the Surveys........................	76
	7.2	Sorafenib (Nexavar)..................................	76
		7.2.1 Post-Marketing All-Case Survey in Subjects with Renal Cell Cancer	76
		7.2.2 Post-Marketing All-Case Survey in Subjects with Renal Cell Cancer/Hepatic Cell Cancer...............	76
		7.2.3 Findings from the Surveys........................	77
	7.3	Bevacizumab (Avastin)	77
		7.3.1 Post-Marketing All-Case Survey in Subjects with Colon/Rectal Cancers...........................	77
		7.3.2 Findings from the Surveys........................	77
	References..		78
8	**Other Molecular-Targeted Drugs (Crizotinib, Alectinib, Etc.)**......		79
	8.1	Crizotinib (Xalkori)	79
		8.1.1 Post-Marketing All-Case Survey in Subjects with Non-small Cell Lung Cancer......................	79
		8.1.2 Findings from the Surveys........................	80
	8.2	Alectinib (Alecensa)	82
		8.2.1 Post-Marketing All-Case Survey in Subjects with Non-small Cell Lung Cancer......................	82
		8.2.2 Findings from the Surveys........................	82
	8.3	Trastuzumab (Herceptin)	85
	8.4	Pertuzumab (Perjeta)	86

		8.5	Palbociclib (Ibrance)	89
		References		90
9		**Antibody-Drug Conjugates (ADC) (Trastuzumab Emtansine and Trastuzumab Deruxtecan)**		91
	9.1		Trastuzumab Emtansine (T-DM1, Kadcyla)	91
	9.2		Trastuzumab Deruxtecan (Enhertu)	94
		9.2.1	Clinical Study (Partially Revised from Reference)	95
		9.2.2	Findings from the Surveys	96
		References		99
10		**Anticancer Drugs (TS-1, Taxanes, CPT-11, Platinum-Containing Drugs, Etc.)**		101
	10.1	Bleomycin (Bleo)		102
		10.1.1	Findings from the Surveys	103
	10.2	CPT-11 (Topotecin, Campto)		103
		10.2.1	Post-Marketing Appearance of Side Effects of Interstitial Lung Diseases	105
		10.2.2	Findings from the Surveys	105
	10.3	Tegafur/Gimeracil/Oteracil Potassium Combination Drugs (TS-1)		106
		10.3.1	Achievement Surveys for Lung Cancer/Other cancers	106
		10.3.2	Findings from the Surveys	108
	10.4	Platinum-Containing Drugs: Oxaliplatin (Elplat)		109
		10.4.1	Achievement Surveys for the Usage	109
	10.5	Platinum-Containing Drugs: Miriplatin (Miripla)		111
		10.5.1	Investigation by the Evaluation Committee of a Third Party	111
		10.5.2	Findings from the Surveys	111
	10.6	Pemetrexed (Alimta)		111
		10.6.1	Findings from the Surveys	112
	10.7	Amrubicin (Calsed)		112
	10.8	Gemcitabine (Gemzar)		112
		10.8.1	Single-Facility Consecutive Surveys	113
		10.8.2	Findings from the Surveys	113
		References		113
Index				115

About the Author

Akihiko Gemma, MD, PhD
President of Nippon Medical School
Professor of Department of Pulmonary Medicine and Oncology, Nippon Medical School Graduate School of Medicine

Biography

March, 1983	Graduated from the Faculty of Medicine, Nippon Medical School
April, 1984	Department of Internal Medicine, Jizankai Medical Research Institute Tsuboi Hospital
April, 1986	Served as a resident in the Pathology Department, National Cancer Center Research Institute
September, 1989	Graduated from Nippon Medical School Graduate School
January, 1991	Served as an assistant of the Medical Office, Nippon Medical School
July, 1991	Served as Chief Physician in the Department of Internal Medicine, Jizankai Medical Research Institute Tsuboi Hospital
May, 1995	Studied at National Cancer Institute, National Institute of Health Laboratory of Human Carcinogenesis
April, 1998	Appointed as Lecturer at Nippon Medical School
October, 2004	Appointed as Associate Professor at Nippon Medical School
	Appointed as Director of Outpatient chemotherapy Unit, Nippon Medical School Hospital
April, 2008	Appointed as Senior Professor at the Department Medicine (Respiratory, Infections Disease and Oncology Division), Nippon Medical School
	Appointed as Professor at the Department of Pulmonary Medicine and Oncology, Nippon Medical School Graduate School of Medicine
April, 2013	Appointed as Dean of Department of Medicine, Nippon Medical School
October, 2015	Appointed as President of Nippon Medical School

Specialized fields, qualifications, official certifications, affiliated committees:
Respiratory Medicine

1. Specialized in the molecular information application for drug treatments of lung cancer, and a co-member in a study which has dictated the individual treatments of chemotherapy for lung cancer (N Engl J Med 2010 Jun 24;362(25):2380–2388).
2. Involved in social strategies for drugs which become problems, in the field of anticancer drug-induced lung injuries which occur commonly in Japanese patients.

Familiar Imaging Modalities:
CT, MRI, PET

Affiliated societies:
American Society of Clinical Oncology
American Association for Cancer Research
The Internal Association for the Study of Kung Cancer
European Society of Medical Oncology
President of the Japan Lung Cancer Society
Councilor of the Japanese Society of Internal Medicine
Director of the Japan Society of Clinical Oncology
Director of the Japanese Respiratory Society
Councilor of the Japan Cancer Association
Councilor of the Japanese Society of Medical Oncology

Part I
Understanding Drug-Induced Lung Injuries

Chapter 1
Understanding Drug-Induced Lung Injuries

1.1 Pathologic Conditions of Drug-Induced Lung Injuries and Factors Inferred from Big Data

1.1.1 Mechanism of Onset

Although the mechanism of onset of lung injuries induced by drugs has not been clearly identified, it has been generally accepted that the pathologic condition occurs through direct cellular damages or indirect ones by inflammatory reactions, an immunological mechanism, by drugs or their intermediate metabolites [1].

1. Lung injuries by direct cellular damages: This occurs depending on the dose of drugs such as bleomycin or busulfan, and the representative cases progress to the chronic stage clinically. In such cases, pathologically, findings of organizing DAD are shown.
2. Lung injuries by indirect cellular damages: The pathologic condition occurs independent of the dose. It is reported that the cases progress to the acute or subacute stage, sometimes to the chronic stage clinically.

1.1.2 Pathologic Conditions

Although pathologic conditions of drug-induced lung injuries are varied, interstitial pneumonia is mainly seen. Pathologic findings seen in interstitial pneumonia drug induced are classified as follows:

1. Nonspecific interstitial pneumonia (NSIP).
2. Eosinophilic pneumonia (EP).
3. Organizing pneumonia (OP).

4. Diffuse alveolar damage (DAD).
5. Hypersensitivity pneumonia (HP).

Generally speaking, the clinical findings of lung injuries correspond to the pathologic ones. But since interstitial pneumonia shows diverse pathologic findings as shown above in i. to v., its clinical picture is varied.

Presently, because studies about image analyses are advancing rapidly, image examination has become an essential diagnostic one for drug-induced lung injuries. Although the findings on images which reflect each pathologic finding are varied, basically, the interstitial shadows explained above are those mainly seen in patients.

1.1.3 Treatments

The basic course of action for drug-induced lung injuries is to first discontinue the administration of the offending drugs and then to conduct oral administration or pulse therapy of steroids as needed. In some cases, an immune suppressor may be administered. Relatively favorable pathologic conditions for steroid treatment are NSIP, EP, OP, and HP. However, in the case of DAD, the reaction to steroids is so poor that it is not rare to rapidly progress to respiratory failure and then to death. Lung injury cases whose course becomes chronic also react relatively poorly to steroids, and even when the administration of the drug is discontinued, the condition may advance and progress to respiratory failure.

1.1.4 Factors Inferred from Big Data

Information about drug-induced lung injuries in Japan has been accumulated through surveys such as post-marketing in-facility surveys and analyses [2]. Drug-induced lung injury in each drug does not always show an identical disease type. While a drug-induced lung injury with any type of pathologic conditions may occur, studies have clarified that the percentages of pathologic conditions of drug-induced lung injuries differ among users of various drugs. In addition, of particular note is that special lung injuries have been reported in users of some drugs. The percentages of pathologic conditions of these disorders and special features of lung injuries are inferred to be caused by the action mechanism of the drug. Information about other risk factors have been obtained, which will be important information used to determine the etiology.

1.1.4.1 Factor 1: Drug

Each drug causes various lung injuries. For example, highly frequent pathologic conditions of lung injuries differ between EGFR tyrosine kinase inhibitors (EGFR-TKI) and mTOR inhibitors. (For details, refer to individual sections.)

1. EGFR-TKI

    DAD appears at a certain frequency and fatalities are relatively high in patients with drug-induced lung injuries. Even in cases where the CT findings at the initial stage show HP-like findings with a ground-glass opacity, some cases shift to DAD as the disease condition progresses. It became obvious that in the initial stage of DAD, the CT images may look like HP in some cases. Figure 1.1 shows cases classified as HP-like or OP-like types by specialist. In Fig. 1.1a the patient condition improved after discontinuation of the drug and steroid treatment, while in Fig. 1.1b steroir treatment was administered but the patient died. As for the difference in results, it is difficult to presume from the situation at the appearance. However, there is a disparity in the history of drug administration: Fig. 1.1a received mTOR inhibitors, whereas Fig. 1.1b received EGFR-TKI. Depending on the history of drug administration, the medical evaluation by physician in charge will be influenced.

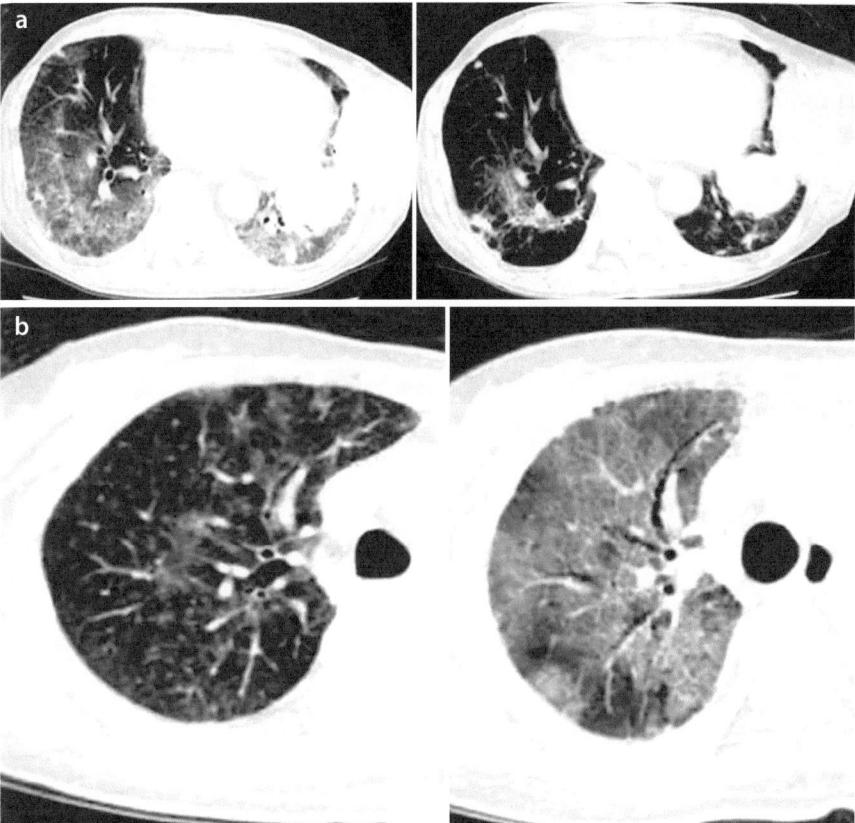

Fig. 1.1 Cases which were diagnosed as HP-like types at the early stage. (**a**) Our case. (**b**) Document provided by specialists committee in enlightening cooperation of the facility (The seventh Japanese Society of Medical Oncology Annual Meeting, 2009)

2. mTOR inhibitors

In cases with HP ground-glass opacities, or the appearance of infiltrated shadows, without any symptoms (Grade 1), the disease condition does not worsen in many cases [3–6], even if administration continues.

Presently, it is difficult to differentiate cases of ground-glass opacity shifting to DAD from cases which remain as the ground-glass opacity. In the situation described above, it was predicted by the features of the drug administered.

1.1.4.2 Factor 2: Personal Genetic Predisposition

It has also been reported that serious lung injuries may be influenced by personal genetic predisposition.

EGFR-TKI induces lung injuries with poor prognosis in many cases; about one-third of Japanese cases. Hagiwara et al. [7] conducted an exome analysis of peripheral blood lymphocytes of patients with acute exacerbation of idiopathic pulmonary fibrosis or serious lung injury induced by EGFR-TKI and compared the results among Japanese, Caucasian, and Chinese cases. As a result, the MUC4 gene[1] was identified. This gene is assumed to be related to the occurrence of a drug-induced lung injury and accountable for the reason why Japanese people are more susceptible for the occurrence of lung injuries than other races. Presently, the polytypic MUC4 gene is indicative as its cause, but future studies such as functional analyses will be necessary.

1.1.4.3 Factor 3: Personal Risk Factors and Organs' Conditions

As a prospective study of risk factors, a case-controlled study was conducted with gefitinib (Iressa) [8]. It was reported that common risk factors between Iressa and other anticancer drugs such as smoking history, pre-existing pulmonary diseases (e.g., interstitial pneumonia), occupancy of the normal lung, age, and systemic condition (PS) are related. As for prognostic factors, age, smoking, pre-existing interstitial pneumonia, and the occupancy of the normal lung which influence the lung condition are also reported . Based on the analysis findings, factors related to the pre-existing lung condition such as smoking history, pre-existing lung disease (e.g., interstitial pneumonia), and age seem to be important as factors of drug-induced lung injuries.

---

[1]MUC4 is membrane-bound mucin developed in respiratory epithelium, and the β chain has an EGF-like domain and acts with ErbB2, ErbB3, and neuregulin to conduct signal communication about cellular survival and proliferation.

1. Smoking history.

    Smoking is listed as a risk factor in the case-controlled study mentioned above and in many other studies. In another study, we conducted an analysis of the *FHIT* gene by the fluorescent in situ hybridization method (FISH method) in idiopathic interstitial pneumonia and reported it in Cancer Research [9]. In pre-existing interstitial pneumonia, it is known that the genetic abnormality causing the cancer had already appeared partially. When this was investigated in the presence or absence of the complicating cancer, the abnormality in the *FHIT* gene was detected in 73% of the cancer-complicating cases and 17% of the non-complicating cases. Because it is reported that the abnormality in the *FHIT* gene is associated with smoking, it may be considered that the gene abnormality is induced by smoking in cases of lung cancer complicated by interstitial pneumonia; therefore, a certain degree of injury may occur in the respiratory epithelium.

    In addition, the abnormalities in not only the *FHIT* but also in *p53* or *Ras* gene are seen in interstitial pneumonia, and it is known that these abnormalities in genes occur due to smoking. Previous injury to the lungs may be assumed in persons likely to have lung cancer, especially smokers. That is, it can be inferred that the high frequency of drug-induced lung injuries in lung cancers may result from a certain level of pre-existing damage causing the gene abnormality in the lungs, compared to other cancer cases.

2. Pre-existing lung diseases (interstitial pneumonia).

    Lung cancer cases complicated by interstitial pneumonia have been investigated in various studies. Undeniably, the risk is high in persons with complicating interstitial pneumonia. The diffuse lung diseases study group in the Ministry of Health, Labour and Welfare surveyed the anticancer drug treatments in lung cancer cases complicated by interstitial pneumonia and reported that the frequency of drug-induced lung injuries differed greatly among patients on different drugs, even among cases with the same level of damage. In the case-controlled study, gefitinib was listed as one of the risk factors for drug-induced lung injuries and especially in patients with interstitial pneumonia, drug-induced lung injuries occurred at a high frequency. In patients with interstitial pneumonia, it is high risk to administer drugs with risk factors [10].

3. Occupancy of the normal lungs, age, and systemic conditions (PS), etc.

    Because the patient's condition fluctuates in the same person and drug-induced lung injuries may more frequently occur with worsened PS or an infection, it is necessary to pay attention to changes in the patient's condition.

1.2 Practice of the Monitoring

In actual clinical use, few clinicians take drug-induced lung injuries into consideration when they administer most of all drugs with monitoring. In cases when a drug with a high risk of drug-induced lung injury is administered or a drug in which a serious harmful event is anticipated, strict monitoring is required. In addition, in patients with risk factors, serious harmful events are more likely to occur and the monitoring method must be thus changed according to the state of the risk. The same monitoring procedure is not always recommended across all drugs and for all patients. Representative cases are presented below.

1.2.1 EGFR Tyrosine Kinase Inhibitors (EGFR-TKI)

It is reported that gefitinib, erlotinib, afatinib, and crizotinib caused drug-induced lung injuries at a frequency of 4–10% in Japan, and 20–40% of these onset cases died [8, 11–15]. In such cases, special monitoring is required. Especially, the disorders are reported to occur at a high frequency during the first 4 weeks after the start of EGFR-TKI administration [8, 11–14]. Thus, it is desirable to monitor the case by chest radiography during the first 4 weeks (minimally, during the first or second week), and subsequently, by chest CT or other imaging technique at an interval of 8–12 weeks in Japan.

In organ cancers other than lung cancer, there are reports that after the appearance of EGFR-related antibodies, the death rate is higher than that seen in lung cancers and the prognosis is poor [16, 17]. In other organ cancers, there is a relatively low rate of chest CT monitoring and ordinary monitoring for tumors is so insufficient that many serious cases may occur. Beside image diagnoses, monitoring by medical interview and chest auscultation is important for early detection.

1.2.2 mTOR inhibitors and Immune Checkpoint Inhibitors

Drug-induced lung injuries occur at a relatively high frequency with mTOR inhibitors such as temsirolimus and everolimus and immune checkpoint inhibitors, but the death rate in all the onset cases is low.

Although CT monitoring was conducted frequently at the beginning, presence or absence of symptoms has become the standard for monitoring because continuous administration is basic for Grade 1 and the post-marketing surveys revealed the safety of this administration method.

Particularly, as for mTOR inhibitors, the safety of the continuous administration for Grade 1 was almost assured by the post-marketing surveys [3]. It is considered appropriate to cope with symptoms at Grade 2, when they appear. However, mTOR inhibitors have an immune-suppressing effect and there have been many reports of infections such as pneumocystis pneumonia [18]. When an interstitial shadow is found, this differential diagnosis must be kept in mind.

With the use of immune checkpoint inhibitors, the appearance of a lung injury around the lesion has also been reported. When a tumor lesion is present in the lung, monitoring should be conducted in the 8–12 weeks after the start of treatment. Imaging diagnosis is conducted within the first month in most of cases. Although continuous administration is standard for Grade 1, the possibility of rapid change in disease condition is similar to that in other drug-induced lung injuries after the appearance of interstitial pneumonia. In the package insert of nivolumab, for Grade 1, administration is discontinued once and its resumption becomes possible. In fact, while observing the symptoms, it is possible to resume administration a short time later at Grade 1. As for pembrolizumab and atezolizumab, the administration is continued with careful monitoring for Grade 1. This difference results from the difference in statements in the package insert. Basically, conditions in many cases allow for continuous administration at Grade 1 [19]. As mentioned previously, it is important to monitor the subsequent symptoms. In particular, because shadows around inflammation or tumors may be enhanced, the monitoring interval must be adjusted, depending on the conditions of the lung [20].

1.2.3 Cases with Risk Factors and Prognosis Factors

In patients with high risk for the occurrence and the severity of drug-induced lung injuries, such as smoking history, pre-existing lung disease (interstitial pneumonia, etc.), the occupancy of the normal lungs, age, systemic conditions (PS) [8], monitoring must be conducted strictly. Depending on the drug used, personal lung conditions, and systemic conditions, it will be necessary to consider the monitoring method on a case-to-case basis.

1.3 Cautions in Interpreting the Big Data Evidence

As stated at the beginning, for new drugs which have an increased risk of drug-induced lung injuries or those for which serious events are anticipated, post-marketing surveys have been conducted in all cases at large-scale facilities. These surveys and analyses revealed the accurate frequency of the diseases, risk factors, and pathologic conditions. These information have been accumulated to be used in proper use of the drugs. However, we recognized some cautions in interpreting these evidence.

1.3.1 Consideration of the Lung Damage

First, it is important to "consider the lung tissues." What is the primary organ of the tumor in the data must be become conscious of. At least, in case of the lungs as a primary organ in the data, the lung tissues, the base for occurrence of lung cancer, are presumed to be damaged to some degree, and the frequency and severity of drug-induced lung injuries may thus become high. For cases in which the same drug is used for other organs, the information obtained for lung cancer must be considered with caution to assess whether the information is appropriate. Conversely, in cases in which the indication increases to include lung cancer, the increase in the severity and frequency must be taken into consideration. For TS-1, irinotecan, and nivolumab, it is known that even among cases with the same drug, the frequency of interstitial pneumonia and the frequency of severe cases may differ, depending on the primary organs [21].

However, in cases of patients with lung cancer, the lung is photographed frequently by CT, and the influence of that monitoring must be taken into less consideration. In addition, the influence may be possible that physicians in charge may observe the respiratory lesions carefully. However, when the information of severe cases are compared, the influence of these carefulness and the frequency of the monitoring are considered only a little. If a difference is present in the comparison of the severe cases, it is considered that the lung conditions have a great influence on the difference. For example, the significant difference in the severity of drug-induced lung injuries demonstrated in the results of surveys in erlotinib-administered cases of non-small cell lung cancer or pancreatic cancer is inferred to be influenced by the lung conditions greatly, although the problem of combined drugs is present [12, 22].

1.3.2 Specificity of the First-in-Class Drug

Next, the specificity of the first-in-class drug must be taken into consideration. In case of a first-in-class drug, the more notable the drug efficacy is, the more patients are waiting for the approval of the drug, so even to the patients whose systemic conditions (PS) are relatively poor, the drug may be administered. Therefore, for the initial situation, these subject patients must be analyzed in detail whether their PS were poor, and necessary cautions must be taken. In taking overall appropriate usage into consideration, this specificity of the first-in-class drug must also be given consideration while the course of the data is checked (refer to the sections on gefitinib and bortezomib).

Expanding the indication to liver cancers, sorafenib (Nexavar) had been used frequently for cases of hepatic dysfunction as a first-in-class drug. Originally, it was limited in Child-Pugh classification and was not used for severe cases of hepatic dysfunction. Because severe harmful events occurred in many patients with relatively poor liver function, based on the findings, a note of that fact was made. In addition, in subsequent reports, it was clarified that severe hepatic dysfunction could occur in patients with change in the liver function detected at an early stage. In the guideline for the appropriate usage, it is stated that patient's medical examination and blood examinations must be repeated at a two-week interval during the three months after initiation of the administration. Careful observation was required such as an examination at week 1. Since the liver is damaged in many cases of liver cancer, hepatic dysfunction is likely to occur. Consequently, although interstitial pneumonia was not noted as a great problem in this follow-up, it appeared frequently in patients with severely damaged liver function.

Although the expert committee for proper usage may offer information about recommended handling, it is very important to collect information immediately after the marketing of a first-in-class drug.

1.3.3 Pulmonary Thromboembolism as Differential Diagnoses

In the Guidelines for the Management of Drug-Induced Lung Disease edited by the Japanese Respiratory Society [23], pulmonary thromboembolisms are not considered to be differential diagnoses. This is because cases in Japanese patients are rare and the disease is classified differently from the classification in Europe and the USA. It is reasonable not to list lung thromboembolism for differential diagnoses for drugs other than anticancer drugs. However, in case of anticancer drugs, because lung embolisms occur in many cases of cancer and angiogenesis inhibitors may be used in these situations, the differentiation of lung thromboembolism must be kept in mind.

1.3.4 Conforming Parameters

The data parameters are extremely important and how the data was obtained must be noted. Although the parameters in all-case surveys are highly reliable information, the data parameters acquired through self-reporting are estimated values and the appearance frequency may become low (refer to the section on erlotinib). Possible variation in the reliability of the results, depending on the data parameters, must be kept in mind.

Because the information presented in this document is not specific to one company, without biased thought to fresh information, this chapter **gives priority not to the newest information but to all-case surveys**. For the newest information including self-reported data, please refer to the homepage of each company.

References

1. Japanese Respiratory Society. Basic knowledge of drug-induced lung diseases. Guidelines for Management of Drug-Induced Lung Disease. Tokyo: Medical View Co.; 2012. p. 1–11.
2. Saito Y, Gemma A. Current status of DILD in molecular targeted therapies. Int J Clin Oncol. 2012;17:534–41.
3. White DA, Camus P, Endo M, et al. Noninfectious pneumonitis after everolimus therapy for advanced renal cell carcinoma. Am J Respir Crit Care Med. 2010;182:396–403.
4. Collective results about harmful events of interstitial pulmonary diseases in achievement surveys of special use of Afinitor® tablets. Novartis Pharma Co.
5. Intermediate report about achievement surveys on specific use of Afinitor tablets (Novartis Pharma Co.) for radical unresectable or metastatic renal cell cancer (From collective cases up to March 31, 2012). http://product.novartis.co.jp/afi/document/.

6. Sun Y, Rha S, Lee SH, et al. Phase II study of the safety and efficacy of temsirolimus in east Asian patients with advanced renal cell carcinoma. Jpn J Clin Oncol. 2012;42:836–44.
7. A study on Japanese specific genetic predisposition involved in acute exacerbation of idiopathic pulmonary fibrosis and drug-induced lung injuries (Study project for overcoming refractory diseases supported by Health and Labour Sciences Research Grant in 2010–2012).
8. Kudoh S, Kato H, Nishiwaki Y, et al. Interstitial lung disease in Japanese patients with lung cancer. A cohort and nested case-control study. Am J Respir Crit Care Med. 2008;177:1348–57.
9. Uematsu K, Yoshimura A, Gemma A, et al. Aberrations in the fragile histidine triad (FHIT) gene in idiopathic pulmonary fibrosis. Cancer Res. 2001;61:8527–33.
10. Minegishi Y, Gemma A, Homma S, et al. Acute exacerbation of idiopathic interstitial pneumonias related to chemotherapy for lung cancer: nationwide surveillance in Japan. ERJ Open Res. 2020;6:00184–2019.
11. Anon. Final report on acute lung injuries and interstitial pneumonia (ILD) caused by gefitinib (Iressa® tablets 250) by specialist committee. Cambridge: AstraZeneca; 2003. p. 3.26.
12. Gemma A, Kudoh S, Ando M, et al. Final safety and efficacy of erlotinib in the phase 4 POLARSTAR surveillance study of 10 708 Japanese patients with non-small-cell lung cancer. Cancer Sci. 2014;105:1584–90.
13. A report on results of intermediate analysis in achievement surveys of specific use of TARCEVA Tablets (Chugai Pharma Co.) for pancreatic cancer (http://chugai-pharm.jp/hc/ss/pr/safe/report/tar/index.html).
14. Gemma A, Kusumoto M, Kurihara Y, et al. Interstitial lung disease onset and its risk factors in Japanese patients with ALK-positive NSCLC after treatment with Crizotinib. J Thorac Oncol. 2019;14:672–82.
15. Information about results of post-marketing surveys of XALKORI® (Pfizer Co.) (March 25, 2013). http://pfizerpro.jp/cs/sv/lc-pro/safety/c_safety_info.html.
16. Ishiguro M, Watanabe T, Yamaguchi K, et al. A Japanese post-marketing surveillance of cetuximab (Erbitux®) in patients with metastatic colorectal cancer. Jpn J Clin Oncol. 2012;42:287–94.
17. A report of final collective results in achievement surveys of specific use of Vectibix® drip infusion (Takeda Pharmaceutical Co.). http://www.vetibix-taleda.com/t2_3.html.
18. Sugiyama S, Sato K, Shibasaki Y, et al. Real-world use of temsirolimus in Japanese patients with unresectable or metastatic renal cell carcinoma: recent consideration based on the results of a post-marketing, all-case surveillance study. Jpn J Clin Oncol. 2020;50:940. https://doi.org/10.1093/jjco/hyaa062.
19. Anon. A report on results of post-marketing surveys of Keytruda® drip infusion in October. Rahway: MSD Co.; 2017.
20. Sata M, Kenmotsu H, Kuwano K, et al. Interstitial pneumonia induced by Nivolumab for Japanese patients with non-small cell lung cancer: A study on the onset risk factor in preliminary results. In: The 15th Japanese Society of Medical Oncology Annual Meeting; 2017. Abstract No. O3–13.
21. Ito K, Jin Z. Characteristics of and risk factors for interstitial pneumonia due to TS-1(R) capsule administration-case reviews from a drug use results survey on non-small cell lung cancer patients and spontaneous reports. Gan To Kagaku Ryoho. 2015;42:595–603.
22. Furuse J, Gemma A, Ichikawa W, et al. Postmarketing surveillance study of erlotinib plus gemcitabine for pancreatic in Japan: POLARIS final analysis. Jpn J Clin Oncol. 2017;47:832–9.
23. Japanese Respiratory Society. Guidelines for management of drug-induced lung disease. Tokyo: Medical View Co.; 2012.

Part II
Actual Practice in Drug-Induced Lung Injuries of Each Drug

Chapter 2
EGFR Inhibitors (Gefitinib, Erlotinib, Afatinib, and Osimertinib)

2.1 Gefitinib (Iressa)

- First-generation EGFR tyrosine kinase inhibitor.
- Indication: Unresectable advanced/recurrent non-small cell lung cancer positive for *EGFR* gene mutation.

Gefitinib is the first molecular-targeted treatment drug for lung cancers, and because many markedly effective cases were reported in the clinical development step, the drug had been highly anticipated. The drug was approved on July 5, 2002, was put into practice first in Japan, and about 19,000 persons had used gefitinib by December of the year. However, soon after the release, 13 patients died after the appearance of drug-induced pulmonary disease and on October 15, 2002, emergency safety information was released. Subsequently, suggestions that this problem may have resulted from handling at the developmental step became contentious. Later, the appearance of drug-induced interstitial pneumonia was recognized to appear in a frequency similar to that of other anticancer drugs, and a court ruled that the appearance of serious drug-induced interstitial pneumonia at a certain level of probability was not predictable. However, through this history, we have recognized the importance of informed consent about the efficacy, safety, and toxicities in developing subsequent medicinal products.

2.1.1 An in-Cohort Case-Controlled Study in Patients with Lung Cancer as Subjects (Fig. 2.1)

Study period: November 2003 to February 2006.
Subjects: Patients with previously treated advanced non-small cell lung cancer.

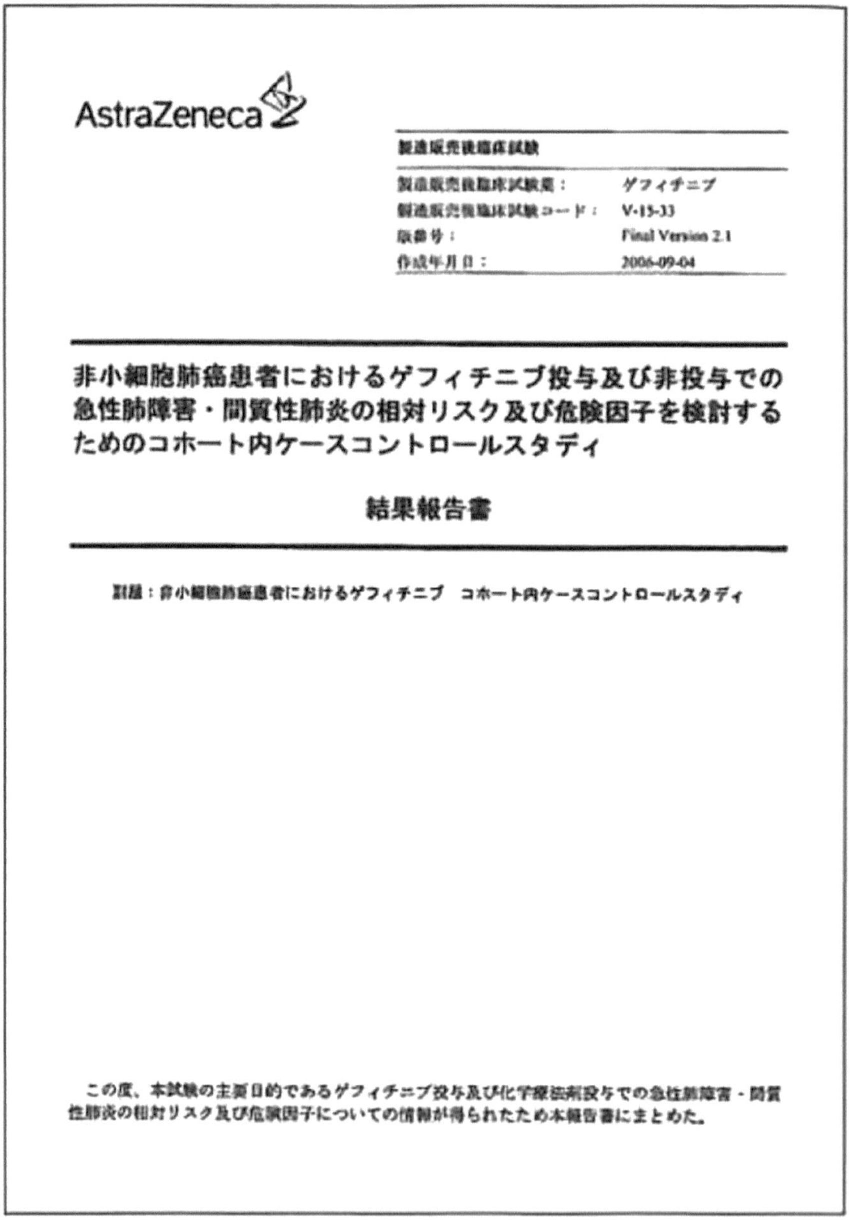

AstraZeneca

製造販売後臨床試験

製造販売後臨床試験薬：	ゲフィチニブ
製造販売後臨床試験コード：	V-15-33
版番号：	Final Version 2.1
作成年月日：	2006-09-04

非小細胞肺癌患者におけるゲフィチニブ投与及び非投与での急性肺障害・間質性肺炎の相対リスク及び危険因子を検討するためのコホート内ケースコントロールスタディ

結果報告書

副題：非小細胞肺癌患者におけるゲフィチニブ　コホート内ケースコントロールスタディ

この度、本試験の主要目的であるゲフィチニブ投与及び化学療法剤投与での急性肺障害・間質性肺炎の相対リスク及び危険因子についての情報が得られたため本報告書にまとめた。

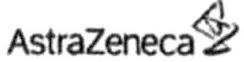

Fig. 2.1 A report on the results of in-cohort case-controlled study to investigate relative risks and risk factors for acute lung injuries and interstitial pneumonia with gefitinib administration and non-administration in patients with non-small cell pulmonary cancer (Cited from Reference [1]

2.1 Gefitinib (Iressa)

Number of subjects: 4473 cases for the cohort registration, 4423 cases for subjects of cohort analysis, 122 cases of interstitial pneumonia, and 574 cases of non-onset.

Observation period: 12 weeks.

Results

Comparison of interstitial lung disease (ILD) incidence: 4.0% in the gefitinib group (95% CI: 3.0–5.1%) and 2.1% in chemotherapy group (95% CI: 1.5–2.9% [2]) (Adjusted odds ratio: 3.2 (95% CI: 1.9–5.4): Table 2.1 [2]).

Fatal cases: 25 of 79 ILD cases in the gefitinib group (31.6%) (Table 2.2 [1]).

Table 2.1 Risk factors of ILD incidence

Explanatory variables	Control	Adjusted odds ratio	95% CI	p value
Treatment	Iressa vs chemotherapy	3.23	1.94–5.40	<0.001
Age	55 years old or older vs 54 years old or less	1.92	0.91–4.09	0.089
PS	PS1 vs PS0 PS2–3 vs PS0	1.57 4.02	0.83–2.97 1.85–8.74	0.001
Smoking history	Presence vs absence	4.43	1.87–10.47	<0.001
Period from the initial diagnosis of NSCLC to ILD occurrence	0.5—Less than 1 year vs less than 0.5 year 1 year or longer vs less than 0.5 year	0.65 0.35	0.37–1.14 0.20–0.62	0.001
Complication of cardiovascular system	Presence vs absence	2.44	0.88–6.80	0.088
Severity of existing IP	Mild vs none Intermediate/severe vs none	4.80 5.55	1.83–12.63 1.40–21.99	<0.001
Severity of existing lung emphysema	Mild vs none Intermediate vs none Severe vs none	1.57 1.04 0.47	0.89–2.79 0.49–2.23 0.16–1.40	0.141
Occupancy of the normal lungs	10–50% vs 60–100%	7.22	2.52–20.64	<0.001

(Based on Reference [2])

Table 2.2 Prognosis in ILD cases

	Iressa (n = 79)	Chemotherapy (n = 43)	Total (n = 122)
Death	25 cases (31.6%)	12 cases (27.9%)	37 cases (30.3%)
Survival	54 cases (68.4%)	31 cases (72.1%)	85 cases (69.7%)

(Based on Reference [1])

Risk factors: Smoking, pre-existing lung diseases (e.g., interstitial pneumonia), the occupancy of the normal lungs, age, and performance status (PS), and administration of gefitinib as a drug-related factor (Table 2.1).

Prognosis factors: Age, smoking, existing interstitial pneumonia, less than 50% of the occupancy of the normal lungs (found on the CT images before treatment), 50% or more of respiratory limited movement area (found on the CT images before treatment).

Time of onset: During the first 4 weeks in many cases.

Topic

First prospective integrated large-scale surveys about drug-induced lung injuries (Fig. 2.1).

For the purpose of prospective integrated large-scale surveys about drug-induced lung injuries, a cohort and nested case-control study was conducted with 3166 cases. The survey is considered the first prospective multidisciplinary joint study about drug-induced harmful events by researchers in the fields of clinical oncology, pulmonary medicine, medical diagnostic radiology, clinical epidemiology, pharmacokinetics, and molecular biology. In addition, pathologic conditions of drug-induced lung injuries associated with gefitinib and the guiding principles for management of the side effects were presented.

2.1.2 Findings from the Surveys

Topic

Special cautions for first-in-class drugs: Large number of use cases, use in PS poor cases.

As for the cumulative course of the appearance of gefitinib-induced lung injuries, ILD appears in over 350 cases during the first four half-year periods and death occurred in about the half of all the cases (Fig. 2.2). During the fourth half-year period of 2006 after the case control study was reported, ILD appeared in about 40 cases and the death rate decreased to about 20–30%.

As for the course, because the patients and their families strongly desired to use the first-in-class drug like gefitinib immediately after its release, the drug was used for patients with poor prognosis or poor PS and the number of use cases thus tends to become high. With epoch-making drugs, it must be kept in mind that harmful events are more likely to occur.

2.1 Gefitinib (Iressa)

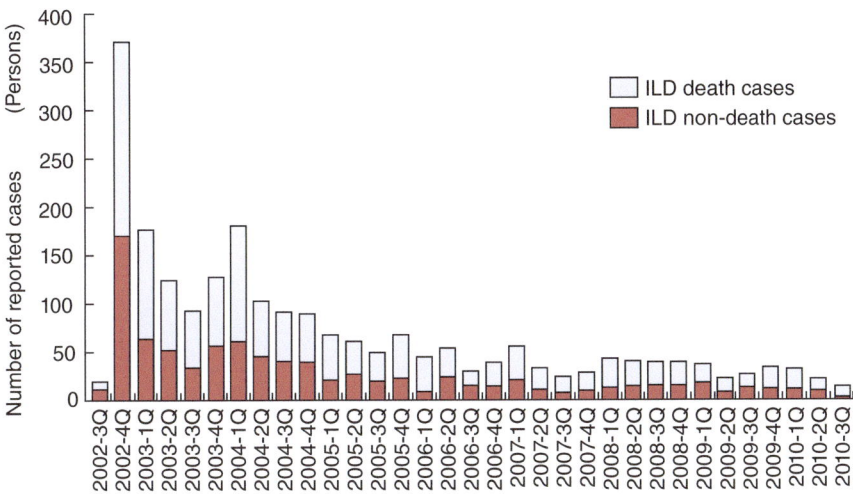

Fig. 2.2 The number of reported ILD cases and the number of fatal cases in reports associated with acute lung injuries and interstitial pneumonia after administration of gefitinib (Aggregated data in individual four half-year periods reported on September 30, 2010). (Cited from the Health, Labour and Welfare Ministry: https://www.mhlw.go.jp/stf/shingi/2r9852000000xthf-att/z2r9852000000xwpk.pdf)

Topic

Attention to the existing condition of lungs in death cases in the interim reports (Fig. 2.3) [3].

At the beginning, 79 cases of interstitial pneumonia collected rapidly by company were investigated. From this data, it was found that there were many death cases having existing interstitial pneumonia. At that time, in image-analyzed cases before the appearance of drug-induced lung injuries, the fatality rates were 75.0% (9 of 12 cases) in cases of existing ILD and 34.8% (23 of 66) in cases of nonexisting ILD (Fig. 2.4) [3]. Specialists of cancer chemotherapy felt afresh the importance of findings indicating pre-existing mild interstitial pneumonia in the lungs.

Inside Story

Dream drug: Highly publicized unexpected side effects.

Because the emergency safety information was announced on October 15, 2002 and it was desired to establish the risk management system as soon as possible, the first expert committee was held on December 5, 2002. The committee decided to

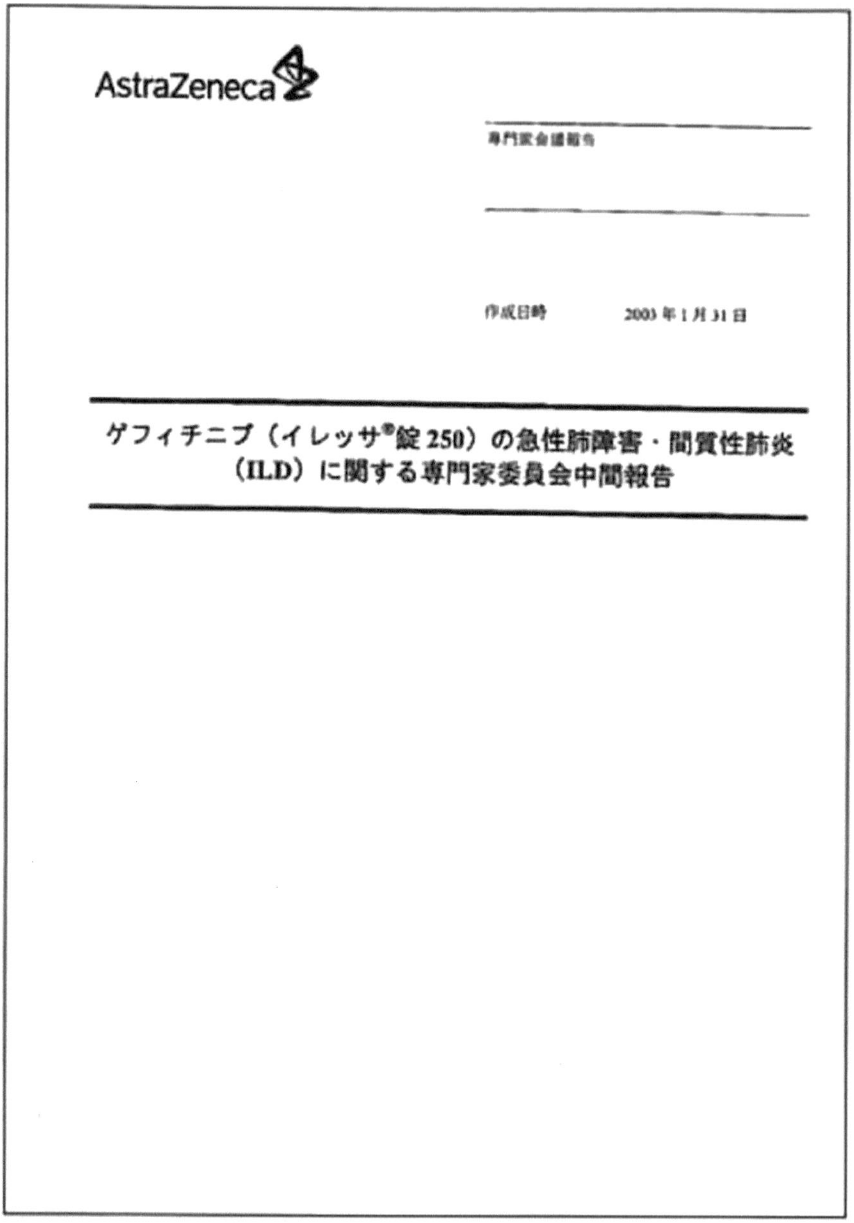

AstraZeneca

専門家会議報告

作成日時 2003年1月31日

ゲフィチニブ（イレッサ®錠250）の急性肺障害・間質性肺炎（ILD）に関する専門家委員会中間報告

Fig. 2.3 An interim report on acute lung injuries and interstitial pneumonia (ILD) induced by gefitinib (Iressa® Tablets 250) by expert committee

present the interim report by the end of January. Soon, 79 cases of interstitial pneumonia collected by AstraZeneca were investigated. Dr. Fumikazu Sakai, Dr. Takeshi Johkoh, Dr. Masahiko Kusumoto, and Dr. Akinobu Yoshimura and I explored the cases.

2.1 Gefitinib (Iressa)

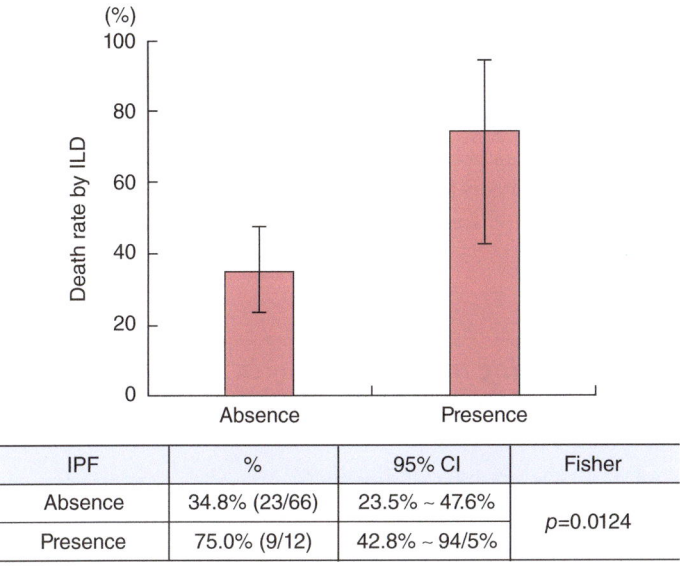

IPF	%	95% CI	Fisher
Absence	34.8% (23/66)	23.5% ~ 47.6%	p=0.0124
Presence	75.0% (9/12)	42.8% ~ 94/5%	

Fig. 2.4 Mortality with ILD in difference of IPF presence and absence before administration of gefitinib (Cited from Reference [3])

In the first report to prescribing doctors on January 31, 2003, it was reported that the image and pathologic findings revealed diffuse alveolar damage (DAD) in death cases and ILD prognosis factors were male, existing ILD, smoking history, and squamous cell carcinoma (Fig. 2.4) [3]. Moreover, subsequent information from study reports and analysis results was provided continuously [2], including the final report by the expert committee on March 26, 2003 [4], the results and discussion about the prospective surveys (special surveys) in August 2004, and the report on the in-cohort case-control study.

Afterward, gefitinib proved to be highly effective drug for mutant tumors of the *EGFR* gene [5–7]. Positively, the main group having the risk factors of drug-induced lung injuries was regarded unlikely to become the subjects for the administration.

Inside Story

Sharing the problem of drug-induced lung injuries in Japan [5].

Globally, there was a difference in the number of reported cases of drug-induced lung injuries among surveyed areas. That is, because the frequency of this event in Europe and the USA is low, it is difficult to obtain an international understanding of the event where a high frequency of cases has been seen in Japan. Thus, in terms of risk management, it became important to obtain the understanding of it. The emergency meeting was held in Seattle, USA, and the special topic of "Interstitial Pneumonia in Patients With Non-Small Cell Lung Cancer," including the outline of the meeting, was published in the *British Journal of Cancer* [8].

2.2 Erlotinib (Tarceva)

- First-generation EGFR thyroxine-kinase inhibitors.
- Indication: Unresectable recurrent/advanced non-small cell lung cancers which got worse after the cancer chemotherapy, and inoperative or recurrent/advanced non-small cell lung cancers positive for the EGFR gene mutation in chemotherapy-naïve patients and (only for 25-mg and 100-mg tablets) unresectable pancreatic cancers.

2.2.1 Post-Marketing all-Case Survey in Patients with Non-small Cell Lung Cancer

Study period: December 2007–October 2009.
Subjects: Patients with non-small cell lung cancer.
Number of subjects: 10,708 cases (9909 cases for the safety analyses).
Observation period: 12 months.
Results: References [9, 10].
ILD incidence: 4.3% (429 cases), 2.6% (257 cases) in Grades 3 and 4 and 2.5% (153 cases) in Grade 5.
Mortality in ILD appearing cases: 35.7%.
Risk factors: Existing ILD/COPD, lung infections, smoking, and period up to the treatment.
Risk factors involved in death: Poor systemic conditions, less occupancy of the normal lungs, and the history of interstitial pneumonia.

Topic

Post-marketing all-case survey of over 10,000 cases [9, 10].

Because the frequency of adverse drug reactions in antitumor drugs is relatively high, the post-marketing survey usually identifies the problem from 2000 to 3000 cases. However, in case of erlotinib, because it had the same mode of action as gefitinib, which had much publicity about the drug-induced lung injuries, and adverse events reported at the time of the clinical trial were also similar as gefitinib, a large-scale all-case survey with 10,708 subjects was carried out (Fig. 2.5) [9, 10]. The reasons why such careful surveys were conducted were because the drug was approved while the contentious matter related to gefitinib was progressing and because there were newly coming up matters in the contestation and the collection of the information about the surveys thus had to become groped.

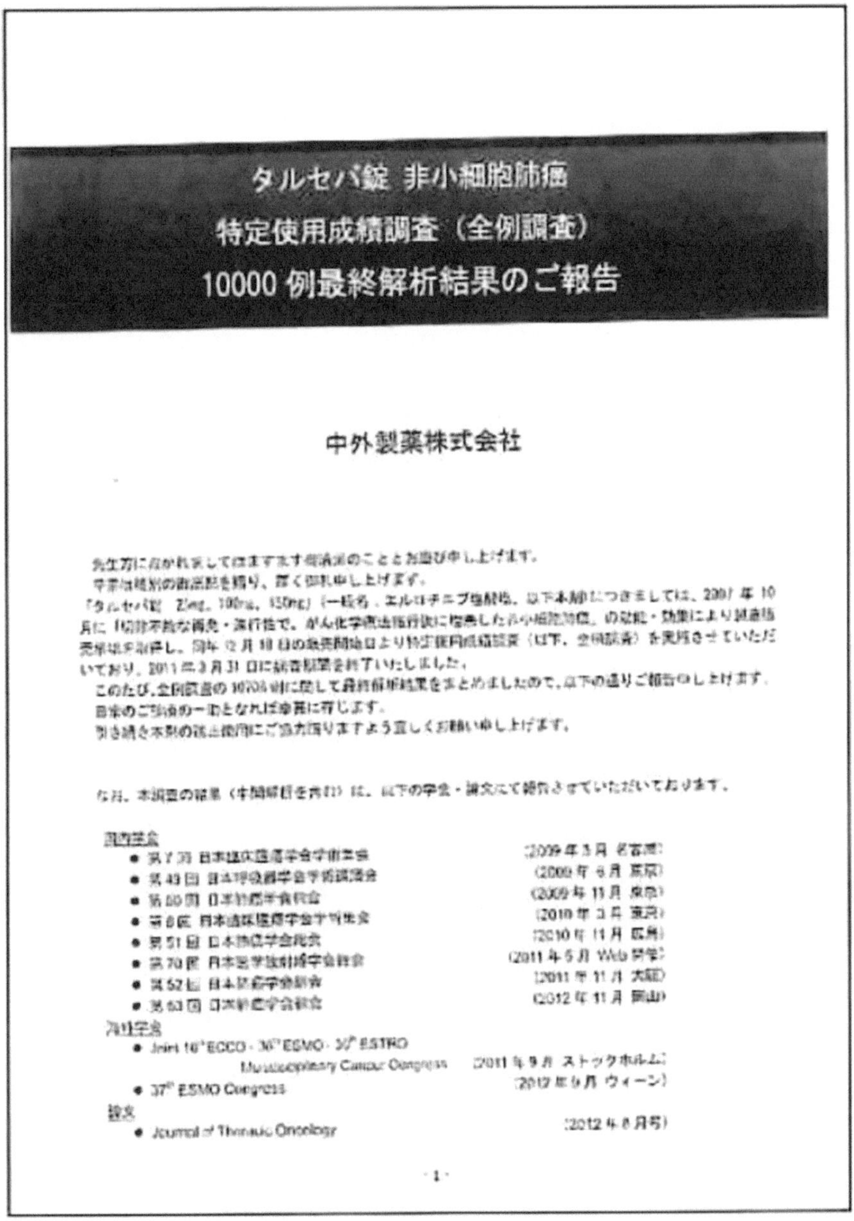

タルセバ錠 非小細胞肺癌
特定使用成績調査（全例調査）
10000 例最終解析結果のご報告

中外製薬株式会社

- 1 -

Fig. 2.5 Tarceva tablets: A report on the final results of 10,000 cases in specific survey of its use achievement for non-small cell lung cancer (all-case survey) in August 2012

2.2.2 Findings from the Survey

Since the drug's action mechanism is similar to that of gefitinib, the adverse drug reactions and risk factors are also similar as assumed.

The management strategies and the surveys of erlotinib-induced lung injuries revealed some specific points. The points are discussed below.

Topic

The occurrence situation differs from that of the first-in-class drug (gefitinib).

Erlotinib was approved after launching the first-in-class drug (gefitinib) and was not used widely immediately after its launching. Consequently, the occurrence of the adverse drug reactions differed from that of gefitinib (Fig. 2.6). The graph shows the cumulative course. By the third month after its launch, there were 72 cases of lung injuries and 19 fatal cases, whose numerical values were close to those of gefitinib at the four half-year periods in 2006 after the results of the case-control study about gefitinib were reported. Thus, the situation with erlotinib could be said to have been stable.

Topic

The methods of big data collection are important: The changing rate of events submitted for the all-case survey during mandatory and volunteer submission periods (Fig. 2.6).

In this survey, cases continued to be registered for a time after the mandatory submission period of the survey ended. Despite the data from over 10,000 cases were accumulated during this period, the numerical values of the incidence of the drug-induced lung injuries and the mortality tended to decrease quickly (Fig. 2.6). The reason for the variation was inferred because only the registration of the cases was required for a period of time, and the mandatory reporting was not required. This indicates the importance of considering the influence of the circumstances of collecting the big data, such as the degree of certainty of the parameter and the reporting situation (for details, refer to the general statement).

2.2.3 Specific Survey of Use Achievement in Patients with Pancreatic Cancer (All-Case Survey) (Fig. 2.7)

Study period: January 2011–August 2012.

Subjects: Patients with pancreatic cancer receiving therapy combined with gemcitabine.

Number of counted subjects: 848 cases (843 cases for the safety analyses).

Observation period: January 2011–December 2013.

2.2 Erlotinib (Tarceva)

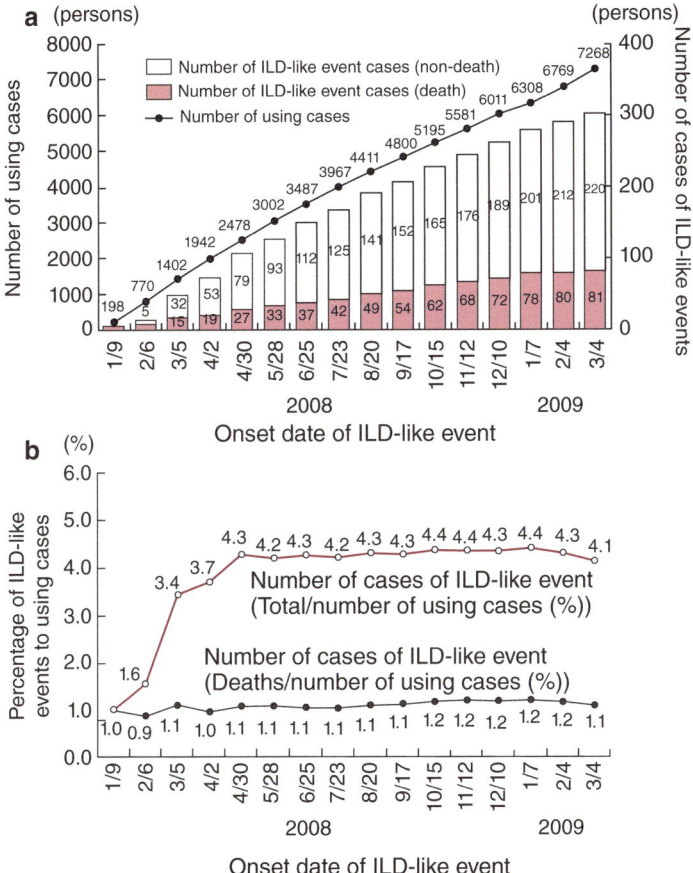

Fig. 2.6 Variation in the incidence of ILD-like events (Aggregated data by evaluation of physicians in charge, at the time on March 4, 2009)

Results: Reference [11].

ILD incidence: 6.16% (52 cases), 2.37% (20 cases) in Grade 3 or severer, and 0.23% (2 cases) in Grade 5.

Mortality of ILD appearance cases: 3.8% (2 cases).

Risk factors: Cases of three or more metastasis, cases of complicated pulmonary fibrosis, and history of interstitial pulmonary inflammation.

2.2.4 Findings from the Survey

Topic

Difference in the occurrence situation between pancreatic cancer and lung cancer: Involvement of the pre-existing conditions of the lung [11, 12] (Fig. 2.7)

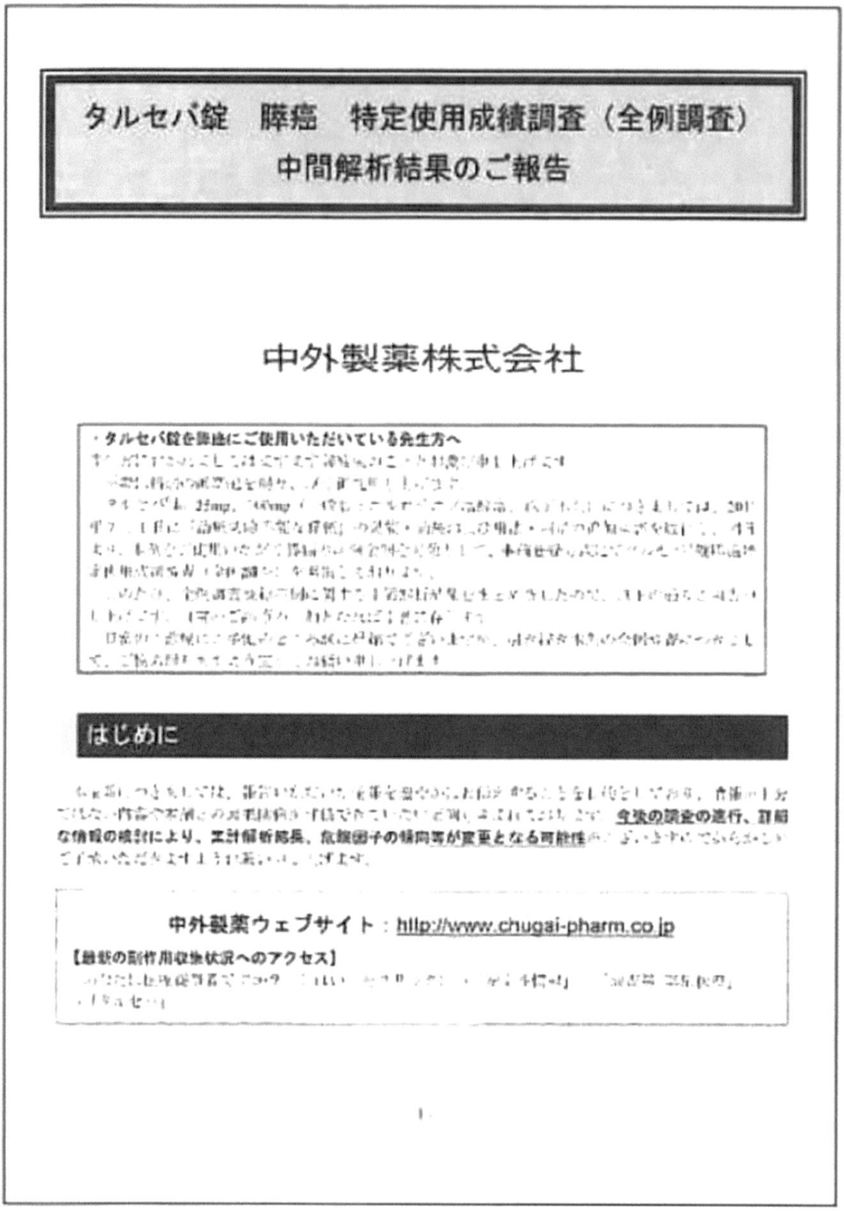

タルセバ錠　膵癌　特定使用成績調査（全例調査）
中間解析結果のご報告

中外製薬株式会社

・タルセバ錠を膵癌にご使用いただいている先生方へ

はじめに

今後の調査の進行、詳細な情報の検討により、集計解析結果、危険因子の傾向等が変更となる可能性

中外製薬ウェブサイト：http://www.chugai-pharm.co.jp
【最新の副作用収集状況へのアクセス】

Fig. 2.7 Tarceva tablets: A report on the results of the interim analysis in the specific survey of use achievement in pancreatic cancer (all-case survey)

- The final ILD incidence was 6.16%, higher than that of lung cancer (4.33%).
- What is most notable is the prognosis after its appearance: Among the patients with ILD, the mortality was 3.8% in patients with pancreatic cancer and 35.7%

in patients with lung cancer, a clear difference. The overall mortality (Grade 5) was 0.23% in pancreatic cancer patients and 1.54% in lung cancer patients, being higher in patients with lung cancer.
- As its factors:
  - The lungs may have more pre-existing damage in the patients with lung cancer.
  - In cases of patients with pancreatic cancer, because gemcitabine in which the ILD's prognosis becomes better than erlotinib is combined, although the incidence is higher, the prognosis may become favorable.
  - It is inferred that physicians have a better understanding from e-learning (refer to the supplementary note), and the selection of the cases and their handling may have been conducted more carefully.

Supplementary Note

Introduction of facilities' and users' criteria in pancreatic cancer: e-learning.
Although erlotinib is indicated for pancreatic cancer as well as non-small cell lung cancer, patients with pancreatic cancer may receive examinations by physicians specializing in lung diseases less often than patients with lung cancer. Thus, an e-learning system has been developed and introduced, available for use by any physician who completed the learning. Presently, the system can be linked up with the facilities' and users' questions shown in the Optimal Clinical Use Guidelines.

Image Analysis Results

Number of subjects: 84 cases of patients using erlotinib in which the image patterns could be investigated.
Results: See Reference [13].
45 cases of faint infiltration, 11 cases of AIP patterns, and 28 other cases.
Among the faint infiltration cases, over 30% (16 of 45 cases) died.
However, this is data of non-small cell lung cancer and it differs from pancreatic cancer (Refer to the topics "Difference in the Occurrence Situation Between Pancreatic Cancer and Lung Cancer").

2.2.5 Findings from the Survey

Topic

Cases with faint infiltration are a heterogenous group: Difficulty in handling.
What was unexpected at the analysis even by the committee was that there were over 30% death cases among the cases of faint infiltration, which is considered to usually have a favorable response to steroids and have a favorable prognosis.

Table 2.3 Image patterns of ILD with erlotinib

Pancreatic cancer		
CT findings	ILD appearance cases (19 cases)	Fatality cases
DAD-like pattern	1	0 (0%)
Non-DAD-like pattern	18	2 (11.1%)
Non-small cell lung cancer		
CT findings	ILD appearance cases (283 cases)	Fatality cases
DAD-like pattern	63	41 (65.1%)
Non-DAD-like pattern	220	71 (32.3%)

(Cited from Reference [13])

As an interpretation of this point, because an early appearance of ILD was assumed from the experience in gefitinib and the follow-up was conducted carefully from the early stage, DAD was detected earlier so that the relationship between the image pattern and the prognosis might be different from typical cases. It is inferred that, along with ordinary faint infiltration, pathologic conditions likely to cause DAD even when treated might be mixed.

In addition, when the image patterns of drug-induced lung injuries were compared between cases of pancreatic cancer and non-small cell lung cancer, the frequency of DAD patterns was notably higher in patients with non-small cell lung cancer (Table 2.3) [13].

Cautions which are summarized up to here are:

- Depending on primary site, the frequency and prognosis of drug-induced lung injuries may differ.
- The cumulative situation of the drug-induced ILD cases may differ between the first-in-class drug and other drugs. As for the first-in-class, particularly cautious must be paid at the beginning after its launching, and cases of faint infiltration include early pathologic conditions of DAD.

2.3 Afatinib (Gilotrif)

- Second-generation EGFR tyrosine kinase inhibitors.
- Indications: Inoperability or recurrent non-small cell lung cancer positive for the EGFR gene mutation.

2.3.1 Post-Marketing All-Case Survey in Subjects with Non-small Cell Lung Cancer

Study period: April 2014–March 2015.
  Subjects: Patients with non-small cell lung cancer.

Number of subjects: 1602 cases.
Observation period: 35.5 days.
Results: See Reference [15].
ILD incidence: 4.4% (70 cases) (3.7% [60 cases] evaluated by the evaluation committee).
Mortality (Grade 5): 0.7% (12 cases).
Risk factors[1]: Male, smoker, PS 2 or higher, complicated lung infection or history, cardiovascular complication, and appearance of an ILD-like event.
Onset time: Appearing within 4 weeks after administration in 76.1% cases.

2.3.2 Findings from the Survey

The incidence and the mortality were similar as gefitinib and erlotinib.
Specific points in afatinib are discussed below.

Topic

Selection bias of treatment-line cases.
With this drug, a favorable response rate after administration of other EGFR-TK1 was found in about 20% cases. This drug has a slightly stronger effect than the first generation of EGFR-TK1 and has wider effect spectrum. However, the results of the post-marketing surveys revealed diarrhea in 78% cases (15% in Grades 3 and 4), which must be considered as another adverse drug reaction besides drug-induced lung injury. Many prescribing doctors have administered afatinib in patients with favorable systemic conditions. For patients who may be susceptible to diarrhea, the first-generation EGFR-TK1 drug was administered. The results of the post-marketing all-case surveys of afatinib showed the presence of a bias reflecting the use in this circumstance.

2.4 Osimertinib (Tagrisso) (Fig. 2.8)

- Third-generation EGFR tyrosine kinase inhibitor, effective against the T790M mutation.
- Indications: Inoperability or recurrent non-small cell lung cancer positive for the EGFR gene mutation.

---

[1] Depending on the number of cases, multivariate analysis was impossible and in such cases, single variate analysis was conducted.

Fig. 2.8 Agrisso® Tablets 40 mg Tagrisso® Tablets 80 mg Achievement survey of use Final report/Results report. (Cited from Reference [14])

2.4.1 Post-Marketing All-Case Survey in Subjects with Non-small Cell Lung Cancer

Study period: March 2016–August 2018.
Subjects: Patients with non-small cell lung cancer.
Number of subjects: 3629 cases (3578 cases for the safety analysis).
Observation period: 1 year.
ILD incidence: 6.8% (245 cases), 2.9% in Grade 3 or more severe (104 cases) [15, 16], 0.8% in Grade 5 (29 cases).
Onset time: 63 days in median value (range: 5–410 days).
Analyses of the image patterns by ILD expert committee.
Subjects: 231 cases which were considered to be ILD.
Results: Reference [17].
11.7% for DAD pattern, 38.3% for light shadow (HP), and 41.1% for organizing pneumonia (OP).
Kushimoto et al. conducted the detailed image analysis shown below, dividing the light shadows into uniform and non-uniform and OP to multifocal patchy and peripheral dominant (Fig. 2.9).
Results: Reference [17].
Mortality: 14 of 25 cases for DAD pattern and 8 of 178 cases for non-DAD pattern.
ILD appearance factors[2]: History of interstitial lung disease and history of previous treatment with nivolumab (Table 2.4).
Risk factors involved in death: History of interstitial lung diseases, history of previous treatment with nivolumab, history of heart disease, and history of lung radiation irradiation.

2.4.2 Findings from the Survey

The onset time tended to be delayed in comparison with other EGFR-TKI drugs.
Among EGFR-TKI drugs, the DAD pattern appears at a low frequency.
The relationship between the image pattern and the prognosis was typical.

Topic

Cautions for interaction with immune checkpoint inhibitors (Fig. 2.10).
Because osimertinib was approved after nivolumab had been approved and marketed, in the post-marketing all-case survey, there were many patients to whom

---

[2] Factors in two types of multiple variate analyses: The point estimation value of the adjusted odds ratio was over 2.0, and the lower limit value of the asymptotic 95% CI was over 1.0.

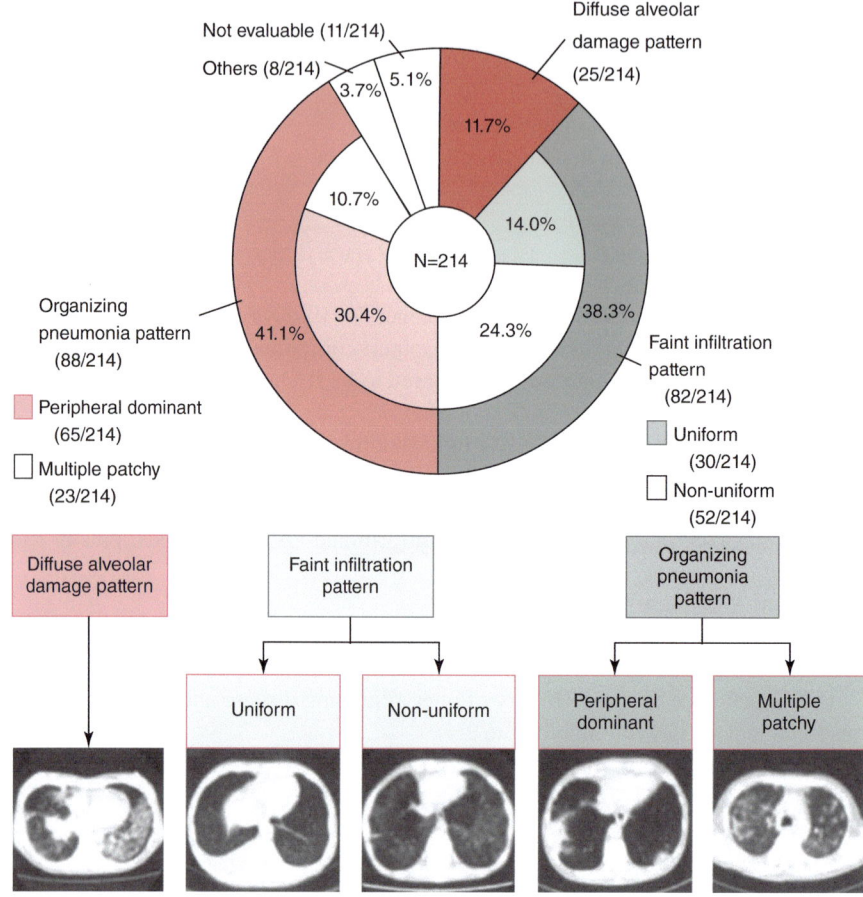

Fig. 2.9 Image patterns of osimertinib (Cited from Reference [17]

Table 2.4 ILD appearance factors and fatal-risk factors with osimertinib

Factors	Adjusted odds ratio (95% CI)
History of interstitial lung diseases: Presence/absence	2.48 (1.98–4.07)
History of previous treatment with nivolumab: Presence/absence	3.51 (2.10–5.87)
Factors	Adjusted odds ratio (95% CI)
History of interstitial lung diseases: Presence/absence	5.55 (2.09–14.80)
History of heart diseases: Presence/absence	4.54 (2.04–10.07)
History of previous treatment with nivolumab: Presence/absence	4.02 (1.62–10.03)
History of lung radiation irradiation: Presence/absence	3.54 (1.42–8.83)

(Cited from Reference [17]

2.4 Osimertinib (Tagrisso)

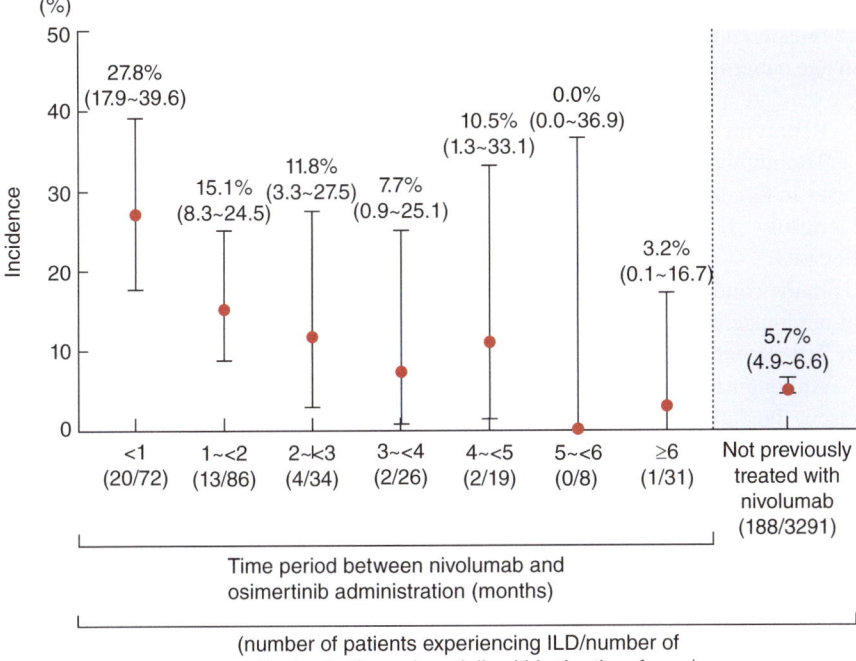

Fig. 2.10 Period after nivolumab administration and ILD appearance with osimertinib (Cited from Reference [17]

osimertinib was administered had previously taken nivolumab. Because it is assumed that the administration of immune checkpoint inhibitors will increase in more patients after chemoradiation therapy or in the perioperative period, the results of the post-marketing all-case survey can be valuable data.

As for the interactions among drugs, although the immune checkpoint inhibitor is considered to have only a minimal influence if the interval is about 5 months after the discontinuation of its use, a shorter interval may have influence (Fig. 2.10). It is necessary to consider other treatments until the administration is switched to the next drug.

Topic

Possibility of re-administration?[15]

Re-administration is not performed when the drug-induced lung injury appears. Although osimertinib is presently used in a first-line (front-line) treatment, the drug was used only for tumor cases with the T790M resistance gene at the time of the surveys. Because there were no other drugs to be administered, the drug was re-administered in patients with mild drug-induced pulmonary diseases, in whom the image pattern of drug-induced lung injury did not indicate DAD. As of March 2021, the data are accumulated.

Report on the re-administration.

The number of re-administered cases: 39 cases (31 cases in Grade 1/2 and 8 cases in Grade 3/4).

Results: ILD incidence: 16.1% in Grade 1/2 (5 cases) and 25% in Grade 3/4 (2 cases).

In the condition that there were no other drugs to be administrated, the drug was re-administered in some appearance cases of mild drug-induced lung injuries. Six of 7 re-appearance cases were Grade 1/2.

Although the judgment is difficult because of the difference with the package insert, the data of the post-marketing all-case survey indicates that the prognosis in some cases may prolong after the re-administration. There have been only a few fatal cases among the appearances of drug-induced lung injuries.

In the future, it will be necessary to investigate accumulated evidence and consider the risk–benefit balance for the improvement of usage. Especially, for cases of T790M mutation, a great benefit may be acquired. However, it is unknown if evidence better than the results obtained from the post-marketing all-case survey will be yielded.

2.5 Vandetanib (Caprelsa)

- Multi-kinase inhibitors targeting VEGFR2, EGFR, and RET.
- Indications: Radically unresectable medullary thyroid cancer.

The ILD appearance in clinical trials in Japan was reported as shown below:

1. Phase I/II studies of subjects with medullary thyroid cancer in Japan: One of 14 cases (Grade 3).
2. Phase II/III studies of subject with lung cancer in Japan: 15 of 125 cases. Three fatal cases were reported (Optimal Clinical Use Guidelines) [18].

Similar to other EGFR-TKI drugs, cautions will be necessary especially for cases with risk factors associated with EGFR-TKI which were reported in the past.

References

1. Anon. A report on the results of in-cohort case control study to investigate the relative risks and risk factors of acute lung injuries and interstitial pneumonia by gefitinib administration and non-administration in patients with non-small cell lung cancer. Cambridge: AstraZeneca; 2006.
2. Kudoh S, Kato H, Nishiwaki Y, et al. Interstitial lung disease in Japanese patients with lung cancer. A cohort and nested case-control study. Am J Respir Crit Care Med. 2008;177:1348–57.

References

3. Anon. An interim report on acute lung injuries and interstitial pneumonia (ILD) with gefitinib (Iressa® tablets 250) by expert committee. Cambridge: AstraZeneca; 2003.
4. Anon. A final report on acute lung injuries and interstitial pneumonia (ILD) with gefitinib (Iressa® tablets 250) by expert committee. Cambridge: AstraZeneca; 2003.
5. Mok TS, Wu YL, Thongprasert S, et al. Gefitinib or carboplatin-paclitaxel in pulmonary adenocarcinoma. N Engl J Med. 2009;361:947–57.
6. Maemondo M, Inoue A, Kobayashi K, et al. North-East Japan study group. Gefitinib or chemotherapy for non-small-cell lung cancer with mutated EGFR. N Engl J Med. 2010;362:2380–8.
7. Mitsudomi T, Morita S, Yatabe Y, et al. West Japan oncology group. Gefitinib versus cisplatin plus docetaxel in patients with non-small-cell lung cancer harbouring mutations of the epidermal growth factor receptor (WJTOG3405): an open label, randomised phase 3 trial. Lancet Oncol. 2010;11:121–8.
8. Camus P. Interstitial lung disease in patients with non-small lung cancer: causes, mechanisms and management. Br J Cancer. 2004;91(Suppl 2):S1.
9. Gemma A, Kudoh S, Ando M, et al. Final safety and efficacy of erlotinib in the phase 4 POLARSTAR surveillance study of 10 708 Japanese patients with non-small-cell lung cancer. Cancer Sci. 2014;105:1584–90.
10. Chugai Pharmaceutical Co., Ltd. Tarceva Tablets. A report on the final results of 10,000 cases in the specific survey of its use achievement for non-small cell lung cancer (all-case survey). August, 2012.
11. Furuse J, Gemma A, Ichikawa W, et al. Postmarketing surveillance study of erlotinib plus gemcitabine for pancreatic cancer in Japan: POLARIS final analysis. Jpn J Clin Oncol. 2017;47:832–9.
12. Chugai Pharmaceutical Co., Ltd. Tarceva Tablets. A report on the results of interim analysis in specific survey of use achievement in pancreatic cancer (all-case survey). http://chugai-pharm.jp/hc/ss/pr/safe/report/tar/index.html.
13. Slides presented at the 54th general conference of the Japan Lung Cancer Society. Speech registered No: 10269.
14. Tagrisso® Tablets 40 mg, Tagrisso® Tablets 80 mg, Achievement survey of use. Final report/Results report. AstraZeneca.
15. Tamura K, Nukiwa T, Gemma A, et al. Real-world treatment of over 1600 Japanese patients with EGFR mutation-positive non-small cell lung cancer with daily afatinib. Int J Clin Oncol. 2019;24:917–26.
16. Ohe Y, Kato T, Sakai F, et al. Real-world use of osimertinib for epidermal growth factor receptor T790M-positive non-small cell lung cancer in Japan. Jpn J Clin Oncol. 2020;50:909–19.
17. Gemma A, Kusumoto M, Sakai F, et al. Real-world evaluation of factors for interstitial lung disease incidence and radiologic characteristics in patients with epidermal growth factor receptor T790M-positive non-small cell lung cancer treated with osimertinib in Japan. J Thorac Oncol. 2020;S1556–0864(20):30717–6.
18. Vandetanib (Caprelsa) (Optimal Clinical Use Guidelines).

Chapter 3
Anti-EGFR Antibodies (Cetuximab, Panitumumab, and Necitumumab)

3.1 Cetuximab (Erbitux) (Fig. 3.1)

- Anti-EGFR monoclonal antibodies.
- Indications: Unresectable advanced/recurrent colon and rectal cancers with RAS gene wild type and head and neck cancers.

3.1.1 Post-Marketing All-Case Survey in Colon and Rectal Cancers (Fig. 3.1)

Study period: September 2008–January 2009 [2, 3].
 Subjects: Patients with colon and rectal cancers.
 Number of subjects: 2126 cases (2006 cases for the safety analysis).
 Observation period: Written in the paper.

3.1.1.1 Results

ILD incidence: 1.2% (24 cases). 0.7% in Grade 3 or more severe (15 cases).
 Fatal case: 10 cases (0.5%).
 Onset time: Period during which the drug-induced lung injuries occur more frequently was not assumed, and the fatality rate was high in cases which occurred within 90 days.
 Risk factors: Elderly persons, patients with a history of interstitial pneumonia.

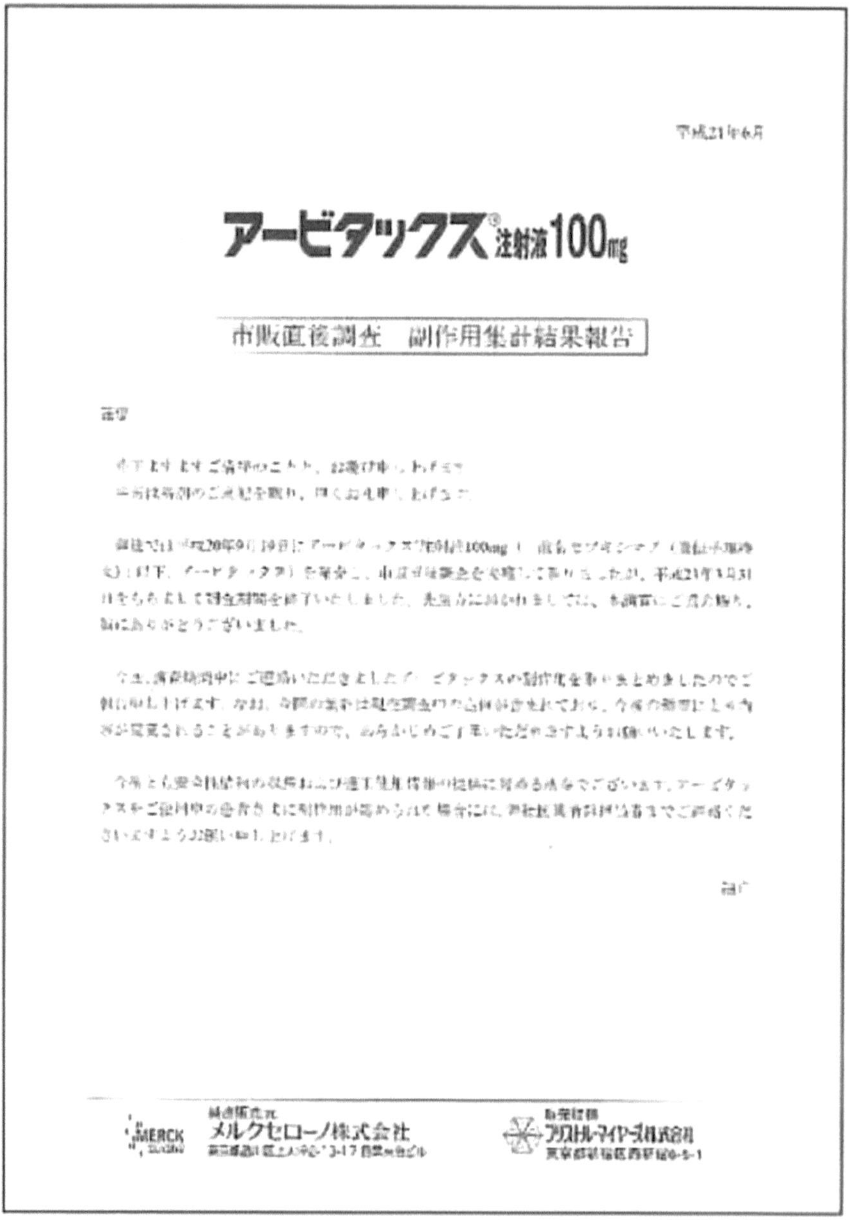

平成21年6月

アービタックス®注射液100mg

市販直後調査　副作用集計結果報告

メルクセローノ株式会社

Fig. 3.1 Erbitux® injection 100 mg A report on the aggregate results of side effect data in the post-marketing survey (Cited from Re ference [1])

3.1.2 Findings from the Survey

Although the frequency of drug-induced lung injuries is low, the population rate of DAD is high (Fig. 3.2). Because the frequency of ILD was similar to that of panitumumab, it may be involved in the effect of the anti-EGFR antibody, but combination drugs for colon and rectal cancer and the medical care situation may influence the risk of drug-induced lung injuries (described later) [1–3].

In this condition, it must be kept in mind that the fatality rate after the onset is 41.7% (10 of 24 cases), higher than those of other antitumor drugs.

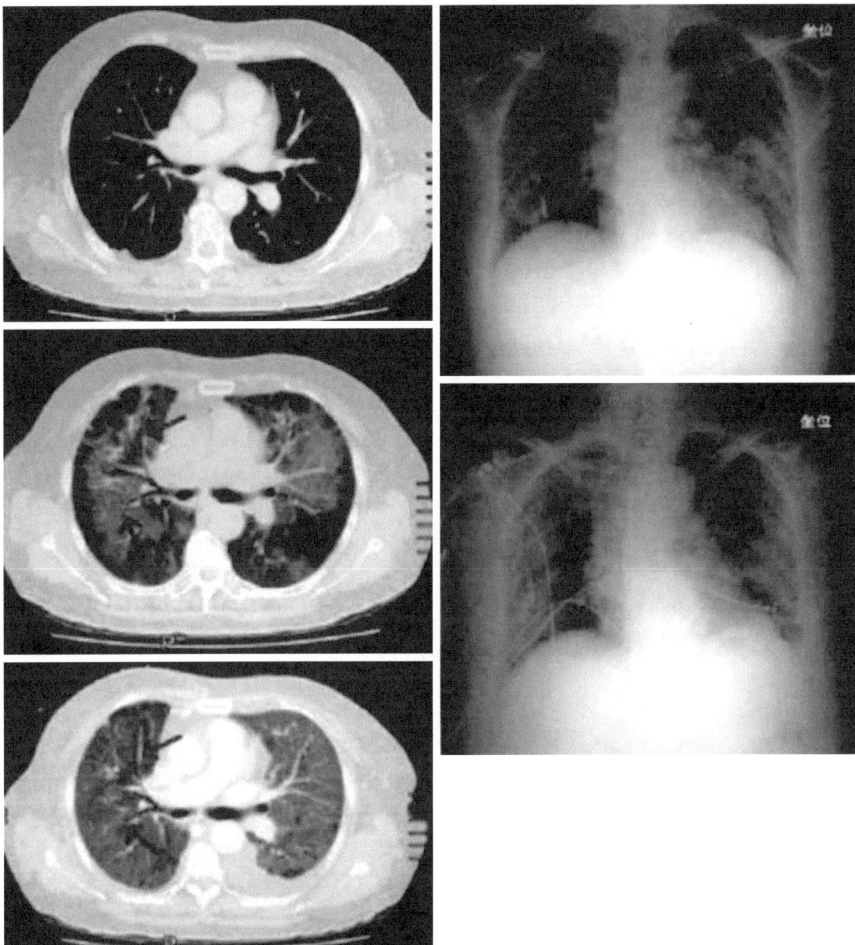

Fig. 3.2 Progress of interstitial pneumonia at the administration of cetuximab (DAD pattern)

3.1.2.1 Topic

Features of head and neck tumors: Frequently occurring accidental swallowing, influence of radiation irradiation.

Cetuximab is also indicated for head and neck cancers. Analyses about this indication have been conducted but not in all-case surveys. Based on the results, the cautions for its proper usage are as follows:

- The incidence of the drug-induced lung injuries in hypopharynx cancer may be high.
- For head and neck cancers, radiation treatment is likely to be administered, and the incidence of the drug-induced lung injuries tends to be high.
- Caution must be exercised for patients with history of interstitial pneumonia (Fig. 3.3).
- Because accidental swallowing may occur in cancer cases of the head and neck regions, when leukocytopenia occurs by other antitumor drugs, it is important to differentiate it from deglutition pneumonia.

When cetuximab is administered, points of caution in head and neck cancers are apparently different from those in colon and rectal cancer. Particularly, caution must be taken for the influence of radiation and the influence on pulmonary events such as accidental swallowing specific for primary organ caused by combined radiation.

3.1 Cetuximab (Erbitux)

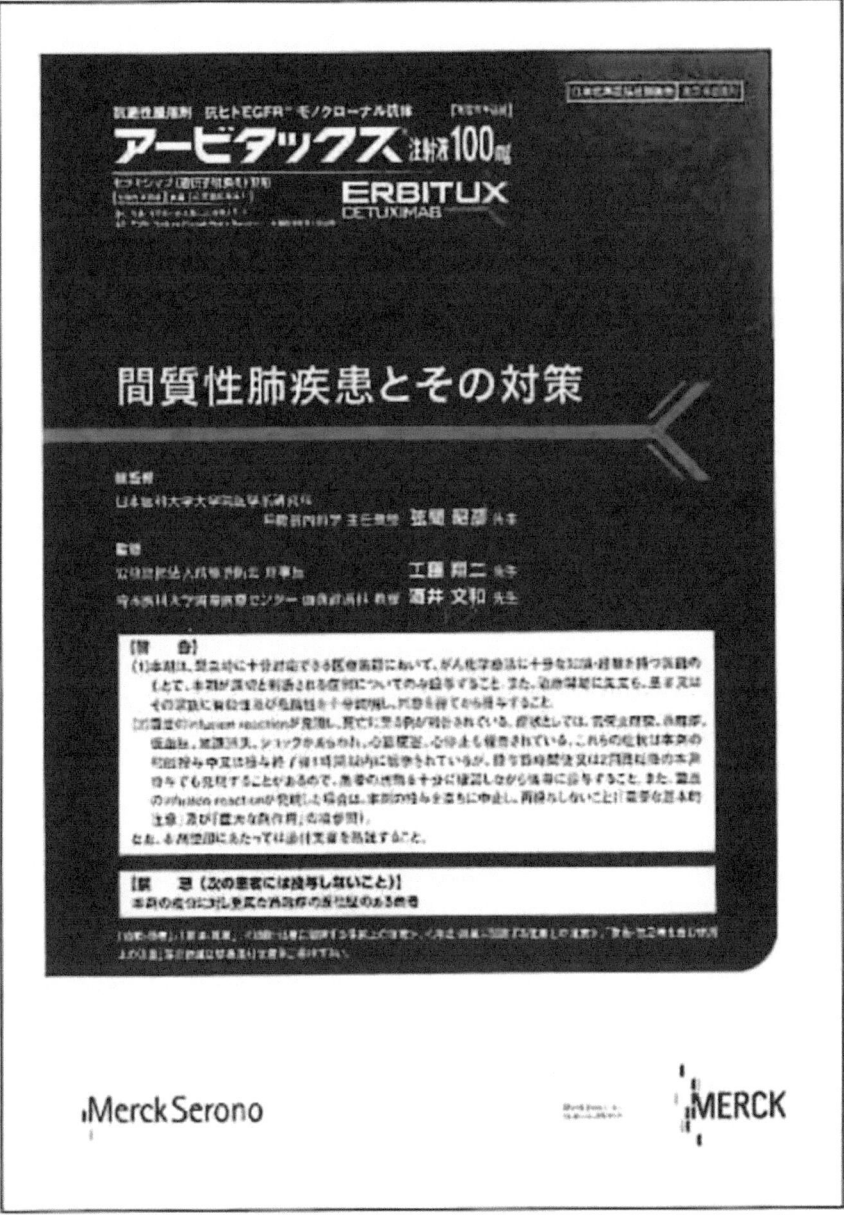

Fig. 3.3 Erbitux injection: Interstitial lung diseases and its countermeasures (Cited from Reference [4])

3.2 Panitumumab (Vectibix) [5–10]

- Anti-EGFR monoclonal antibodies.
- Indications: Patients with unresectable advanced/recurrent colon and rectum cancers with KRAS gene wild type.

3.2.1 Post-Marketing All-Case Survey in Patients with Colon and Rectal Cancers

Study period: June 2010–July 2012.
 Subjects: Patients with colon/rectal cancers.
 Number of subjects: 3085 cases for the safety analysis.
 Observation period: 10 months.
 Results: Reference [5].
 Incidence and fatality rate of interstitial lung diseases: 1.3% (39 cases), 20 cases (0.6%) for the death cases, 51.3% for the fatality rate [5–9].
 Risk factors: Existing interstitial lung diseases, male, poor PS, and 65 years old or older (Fig. 3.4) [9].
 Image pattern (in 39 cases): 18 cases (46.2%) for the DAD pattern (Table 3.1) [9].
 Onset time of interstitial pneumonia: Period during which the disease occurs more frequently was not assumed.

3.2.2 Findings from the Survey

A large-scale post-marketing all-case survey was carried out in about 2000 users of cetuximab and about 3000 users of panitumumab, and almost similar results were obtained with the incidence rate of interstitial lung diseases (1.2%, 1.3%), the fatality rate (0.6%, 0.5%), and the fatality rate after the onset (41.7%, 51.3%). The data can be used to demonstrate reproducibility in drugs with the same drug efficacy.

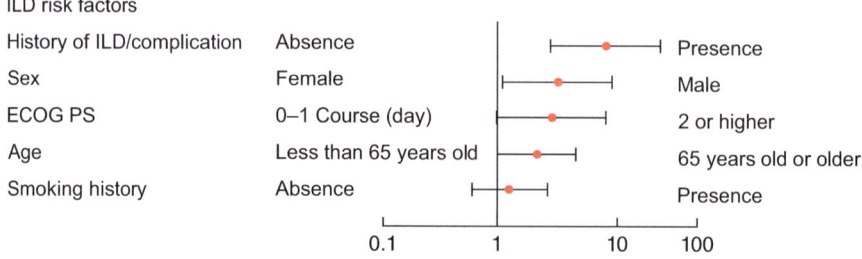

Fig. 3.4 Forest plot of risk factors (Cited from Reference [9])

3.2 Panitumumab (Vectibix)

Table 3.1 Incidence and time of ILD's image pattern

	Total number	Within 1 month	Within 2 months	Within 3 months	Within 4 months	Within 5 months	Within 6 months	Within 7 months	Within 8 months	Within 9 months	Within 10 months	Over 10 months
DAD	18 (15)	4 (4)	1 (1)	6 (4)	1 (0)	2 (2)	2 (2)		1 (1)			1 (1)
HP	9 (1)	1 (0)	1 (1)	3 (0)		1 (0)	1 (0)		2 (0)			
OP	8 (0)	1 (0)	2 (0)	2 (0)		1 (0)	1 (0)			1 (0)		
Unevaluable	4 (3)	2 (2)					1 (0)			1 (1)		
Total number	39 (19)	8 (6)	4 (2)	11 (4)	1 (0)	4 (2)	5 (2)	0 (0)	3 (1)	2 (1)	0 (0)	1 (1)

The values in the brackets indicate the number of deaths. The aggregated data by the image patterns at the final outcome. *DAD* diffuse alveolar damage, *HP* hypersensitivity pneumonia, *OP* organizing pneumonia (Cited from Reference [9])

Frequent image patterns were DAD, and these cases increased the mortality (Table 3.1) [9].

The above description is summarized below:

With cetuximab and panitumumab, the frequency of drug-induced interstitial lung diseases is relatively low and the mortality is high.

Physicians in charge must evaluate the risks with patient's lung conditions and medical history in mind to make efforts for early diagnosis and treatment by careful observation if needed.

3.2.2.1 Topic

Common matters between cetuximab and panitumumab: The problem of a high probability of DAD.

The outlines of the incidence of interstitial lung diseases in both drugs were similar. In the results of the surveys, among cases in Japanese patients with anti-EGFR antibodies, deaths with the occurrence of DAD were shown with reproducibility. As for cetuximab and panitumumab, it is a question that, compared to the results of the all-case surveys for other drugs, the occurrence of interstitial lung diseases was slightly less, but the fatality rate was higher. The inferred factors are as follows:

1. Difference in the observation frequency and methods.

    Before the post-marketing all-case survey for both the drugs, the high rate of the incidence of drug-induced lung injuries had been given special attention when used in patients with lung cancers and chest CTs were conducted regularly as part of routine clinical practice. However, in case of colon and rectum cancer, an indication for both of the drugs, although the frequency of its pulmonary metastasis is relatively high, chest CTs were not conducted on a regular basis in any of the cases. It is presumed that mild interstitial pneumonia, which had been recognized on CT images in the past was overlooked and thus, the incidence of interstitial pneumonia became low. Moreover, because the denominator was small, the fatality rate might become high in appearance. It follows that frequent screenings will increase the possibility for the early detection.

2. Differences in the lung tissues conditions of subjects with disease.

    Because the lung tissues in patients with lung cancer are more damaged, the frequency of interstitial pneumonia in patients with lung cancer may be higher. This point will be explained in detail in other section. Data about drugs used for multiple primary organs including lung cancer such as CPT-11, TS-1, nivolumab, and bleomycin show a higher frequency in lung cancer. However, the absolute number of fatal cases may increase.

3. Presence or absence of combined drugs.

    The third matter noted is the effect of combined drugs. A high number of fatal cases may result from this factor.

    In the final analysis of cetuximab, the presence or absence of combined anti-cancer drugs was analyzed. The mortality was 0.43% (2 of 460 cases) in cases of monotherapy treatment and 1.36% (21 of 1546 cases) in cases with combined drugs, indicating a tendency but no significant difference.

With panitumumab, the appearance rate was 1.3% in both the cases of combined therapy and monotherapy.

However, in the survey of both the drugs, the number of cases noting pretreatment differed in a subtle way; therefore, the effect of presence or absence of combined drugs cannot be easily discussed.

The mortality is considered the numerical value estimated by the balance among the percentage of diagnosed mild interstitial pneumonia and the rate of severe cases. At any rate, when the interstitial pneumonia occurs under these usage conditions, the high mortality must be kept in mind.

3.3 Necitumumab (Portrazza) [11]

- Anti-EGFR monoclonal antibodies.
- Indications: Patients with unresectable advanced/recurrent squamous non-small cell lung cancer.

3.3.1 Post-Marketing Survey in Patients with Squamous Cell Lung Cancer

Study period: November 2019–May 2020.
 Subjects: Patient with squamous cell lung cancer.
 Number of cases with side effects: 21 cases.
 Results: No appearances of interstitial lung disease.
 As for the aggregated number of cases of side effects, because of the positioning of this drug and the usages and doses for combined use of gemcitabine and cisplatin, the case collection was ended with only 21 cases. Among the 21 cases, there were no cases of interstitial lung disease.

References

1. Anon. Erbitux injection 100 mg. A report on the aggregate results of the side effect data in the early post-marketing survey. Supplement interstitial lung diseases. Darmstadt: Merck Serono Co., Ltd. Bristol Myers Company; 2009.
2. Ishiguro M, Watanabe T, Yamaguchi K, et al. A Japanese post-marketing surveillance of cetuximab (Erbitux®) in patients with metastatic colorectal cancer. Jpn J Clin Oncol. 2012;42:287–94.

3. Satoh T, Gemma A, Kudoh S, et al. Incidence and clinical features of drug-induced lung injury in patients with advanced colorectal cancer receiving Cetuximab: results of a prospective multicenter registry. Jpn J Clin Oncol. 2014;44:1032–9.
4. Erbitux injection 100 mg. Interstitial lung diseases and its countermeasures.
5. Osawa M, Kudoh S, Sakai F, et al. Clinical features and risk factors of panitumumab-induced interstitial lung disease: a postmarketing all-case surveillance study. Int J Clin Oncol. 2015;20:1063–71.
6. Boku N, Sugihara K, Kitagawa Y, et al. Panitumumab in Japanese patients with Unresectable colorectal cancer: a post-marketing surveillance study of 3085 patients. Jpn J Clin Oncol. 2014;44:214–23.
7. Vectibix® drip infusion 100 mg. Specific surveys for the usage achievement. A report on the interim aggregate results. Takeda Pharmaceutical Co., Ltd.
8. Vectibix® drip infusion 100 mg. An early post-marketing surveys. Notification of the results. Takeda Pharmaceutical Co., Ltd.
9. Takeda Pharmaceutical Co., Ltd. Specific surveys for the usage achievement of Vectibix® drip infusion. A report on the final aggregate results. Tokyo: Takeda Pharmaceutical Co., Ltd. http://www.vectibix-takeda.com/t2_3.html
10. Vectibix® drip infusion 100 mg/drip infusion 400 mg. Achievement surveys of the specific usage. A report of the second aggregate results.
11. Anon. Portrazza drip infusion 800 mg. A report on the results in the early post-marketing surveys. Tokyo: Nippon Kayaku CO., Ltd.; 2020.

Chapter 4
mTOR Inhibitors (Temsirolimus and Everolimus)

4.1 Temsirolimus (Torisel)

- mTOR inhibitor drops,
- Indications: Radically unresectable or metastatic renal cell cancer.

4.2 Everolimus (Afinitor)

- Oral mTOR inhibitors.
- Indications: Radically unresectable or metastatic renal cell cancers, neuroendocrine cancer, inoperative or recurrent breast cancer, and nodular sclerosis.

Temsirolimus (Torisel) and everolimus (Afinitor) are mTOR inhibitors[1] which were launched at almost the same time. The mTOR inhibitors were admitted first as anticancer drugs for renal cell cancer, and then, the indications with everolimus were expanded to cases of radically unresectable or metastatic neuroendocrine tumors, breast cancer, and nodular sclerosis.

The final data of post-marketing all-case survey in Japanese people is summarized below.

---

[1] Temsirolimus was approved first and everolimus was approved shortly thereafter.

4.2.1 Post-Marketing All-Case Survey in Patients with Renal Cell Cancer

Temsirolimus:
  Study period: September 2010–September 2012.
  Subjects: Patients with renal cell cancer.
  Number of subjects: 1052 cases (1001 cases for the safety analysis).
  Observation period: 24–96 weeks.
  Results: Reference [1].
  ILD incidence: 17.38% (174 cases), 4.50% (45 cases) in Grade 3 or more severe.
  Fatal cases (Grade 5): 9 cases (0.90%).
  Other toxic events: 9 cases of pneumocystis pneumonia, among the cases, four cases died (0.4%).
  Everolimus (Fig. 4.1).
  Study period: Time of product launch—March 31, 2012.
  Subjects: Patients with radically unresectable or metastatic renal cell cancer.
  Number of subjects: 1077 cases (1067 cases for the safety analysis).
  Results: Reference [2].
  ILD incidence: 22.9% (244 cases), severe cases 7.3% (78 cases).
  Fatal cases: 7 cases (0.7%).
  For the latest information including all reported cases as well as the all-case survey, see the website: https://drs-net.novartis.co.jp/dr/products/product/afinitor/.

4.2.2 Findings from the Surveys

No great difference in the fatality rate was found between the drugs.

Similar drug-induced lung injuries were found between temsirolimus and everolimus. When considering if continuous administration in clinically asymptomatic cases is appropriate, in Japanese patients whose possibility of the seriousness is pointed out depending on types of drug-induced lung injuries, it was concluded that continuous administration would be allowable[3], because the post-marketing surveys revealed no deaths among 68 Grade 1 cases with continuous administration, see Fig. 4.2.

Features of both drugs

1. The incidence of interstitial pneumonia (ILD) is high, 20–30%, in both drugs. If mild cases are also followed up, the incidence is assumed to become higher than the reported rate[4].
2. Although the incidence is high, some mild cases have disappeared after continuous treatment and the prognosis has been relatively favorable.

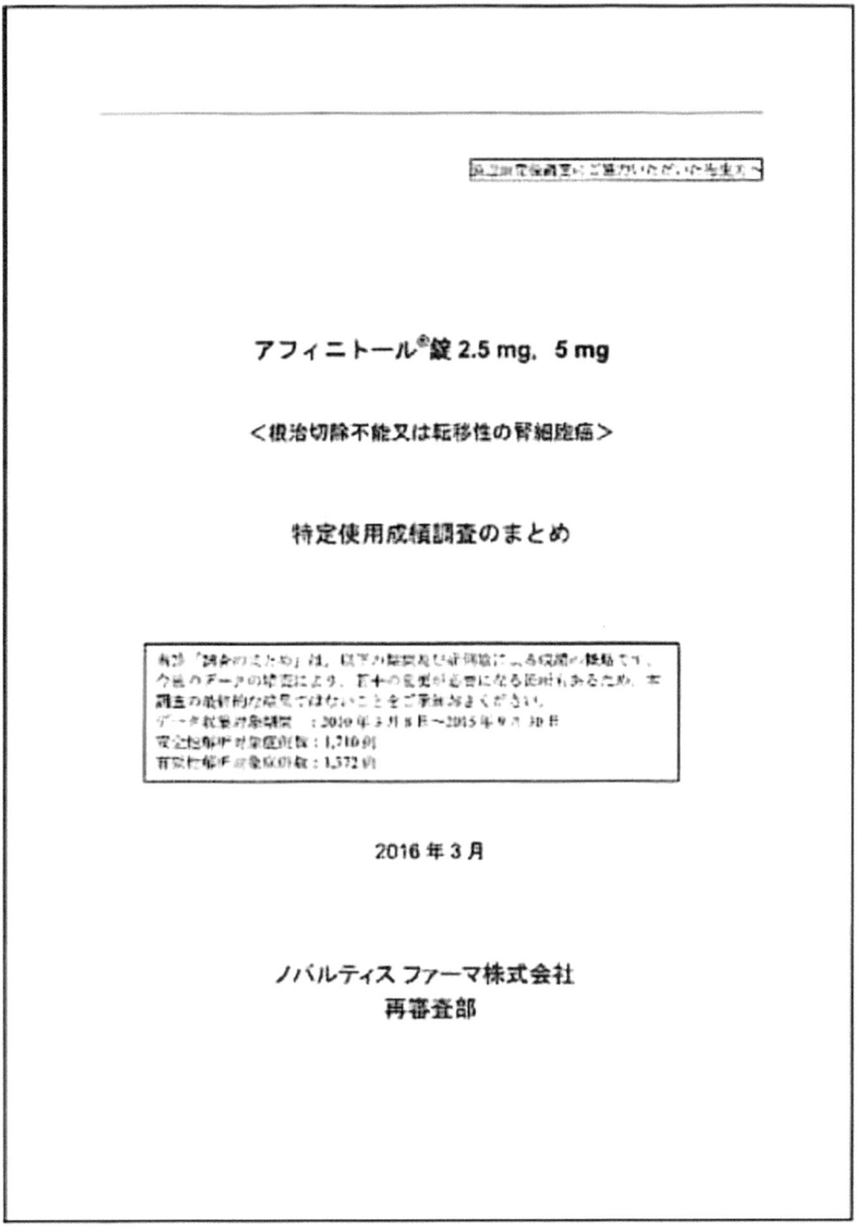

4.2 Everolimus (Afinitor)

アフィニトール®錠 2.5 mg, 5 mg

＜根治切除不能又は転移性の腎細胞癌＞

特定使用成績調査のまとめ

2016 年 3 月

ノバルティス ファーマ株式会社
再審査部

Fig. 4.1 Afinitor® Tablets 2.5 mg, 5 mg < radically unresectable or metastatic renal cell cancer > summary of specific surveys of usage achievement. (Cited from Reference [2])

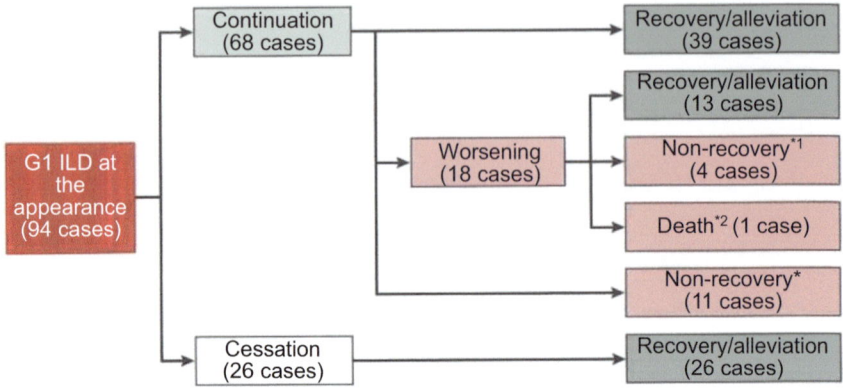

Fig. 4.2 Outcome of G1 cases at the appearance of temsirolimus-induced interstitial lung disease (Cited from Reference [3])

3. Basic image findings are uniform with frosted glass-like shadows and organizing pneumonia (OP)-like shadows (Fig. 4.3).
4. Other than images, clinical findings include a bronchoalveolar lavage (BAL) finding characterized by the lymphocytic predominance (Table 4.1) [5]. The method to cope with this adverse event is to discontinue administration or continuous administration. Because of favorable steroid reactivity, the drug is administered continuously when clinical symptoms are absent, and when a symptom appears, the administration is discontinued.

Notable characteristics of both drugs are shown below.

4.2.2.1 Topic

Was the increase in the biomarkers (KL-6, SP-D) identified earlier than that seen on the images? [2].

In patients with interstitial pneumonia, an increase in the biomarkers (KL-6, SP-D) used in Japan is highly frequent, and the increase is also seen even in many Grade 1 cases (KL-6: 13 of 17 cases) (Figs. 4.4 and 4.5). In addition, among the high cases for KL-6 and SP-D, there are no findings on images in some cases.

4.2.2.2 Inside Story

Handling of Grade 1 cases and monitoring in post-marketing all-case survey of Japanese patients: Specificity of Japanese population should be recognized overseas.

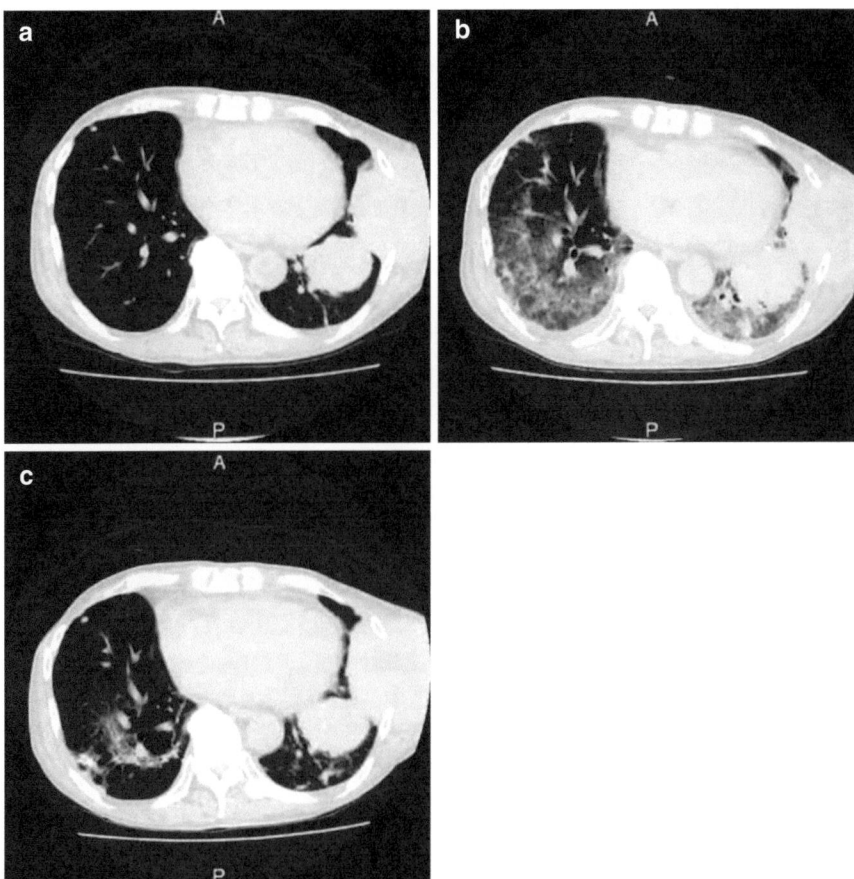

Fig. 4.3 Progress of typical interstitial lung diseases severe case by mTOR inhibitors. A respiratory difficulty occurred. **Non-segmental pulmonary filtrate and frosted glass-li**ke shadows were found. The case responded to steroids favorably and then improved

As my experiences, I would like to introduce about overseas situation and handling in Japan. Previous survey reports about EGFR-TKI have pointed out that the frequency of drug-induced lung injuries and the fatal cases (DAD) tends to be high in Japan. It was considered that careful observation in post-marketing management of adverse drug reactions was necessary because the drug-induced lung injuries were seen at an extremely high frequency. Thus, it was suggested to shorten the interval of the follow-up immediately after the administration in Japan. Although the Pfizer and Novartis initially desired to aimed to establish a single global management guideline, an understanding about the unique Japanese approach in which follow-up is conducted more carefully in Japan, after discussions about the Optimal Clinical Use Guidelines with the company.

Table 4.1 Clinical examination values related to interstitial lung diseases and bronchoalveolar lavage

No.	Names of reported events	Grade	Collected date (day)	Lymphocytes (%)	Neutrophils (%)	Eosinophils (%)	Macrophages (%)	Ratio of CD4/CD8
1	Interstitial lung diseases	2	7	73.7	0	0	26.2	7.35
2	Interstitial lung diseases Pneumocystis pneumonia	5	0	54.7	26.3	4	–	–
3	Radiation pneumonia Interstitial lung diseases	3	3	55.4	0.8	7	35.5	–
4	Interstitial lung diseases	2	1	81.6	1.6	2.6	13.8	–
5	Interstitial lung diseases	2	16	–	–	–	–	16.38
6	Interstitial lung diseases	3	2	20	3	2	75	5.07
7	Interstitial lung diseases	3	9	64.5	2.5	–	23	7.15
8	Pneumonia	2	8	94	–	–	–	12.4

Note: Number of days from the appearance date

Afinitor tablets. Aggregated results of the adverse event of interstitial lung diseases in the specific achievement surveys. 2011 Bronchoalveolar lavage was conducted in 8 cases among the appearances of interstitial lung diseases. The percentage of lymphocytes was high in 6 of the 8 cases. (Cited from Reference [5])

4.2 Everolimus (Afinitor)

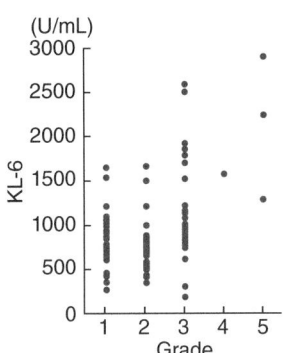

Fig. 4.4 KL-6 values in different grades There were 73 cases among the subjects. Each worst grade was recorded for each case. For KL-6 values, a plot was made of the worst value after the appearance of interstitial lung disease. (Cited from Reference [5])

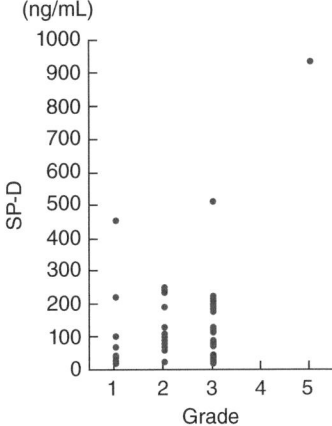

Fig. 4.5 SP-D values in different grades. There were 37 cases among the subjects. The worst grade was reported for each case. For SP-D values, a plot was made of the worst value after the appearance of interstitial lung diseases. (Cited from Reference [5])

Afterward, the topic of whether continuous administration/re-administration in Grade 1 was allowable was also considered.

The results in the cases of continuous administration/re-administration in the past were reported as follows.

With temsirolimus, when continuous administration was conducted in 68 of 94 Grade 1 cases, only one subject with complicated interstitial pneumonia died, and there were no other deaths (Fig. 4.2) [3]. In addition, it recurred in 4 of 27 cases of the re-administration, and then, the 4 cases recovered (Fig. 4.6) [3]. With everolimus, the drug was administered continuously in 68 of 94 Grade 1 cases and no deaths occurred (Fig. 4.7) [2].

Based on the finding that the frequency of DAD is not high as shown in the surveys mentioned above, finally, it was concluded that the same management of toxic events as that used overseas was acceptable. Constantly with the specificity of drug-induced lung injuries in Japanese people in mind, it is considered important to identify risks as early as possible.

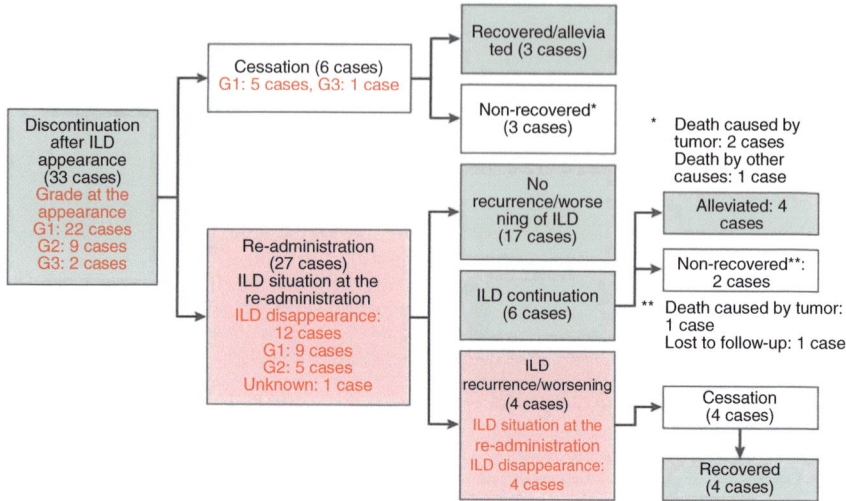

Fig. 4.6 Temsirolimus re-administered cases after the appearance of interstitial lung disease Among 27 cases of re-administration after the administration had been discontinued once after ILD appeared, ILD recurred in 4 cases (14.8%). (Cited from Reference [3])

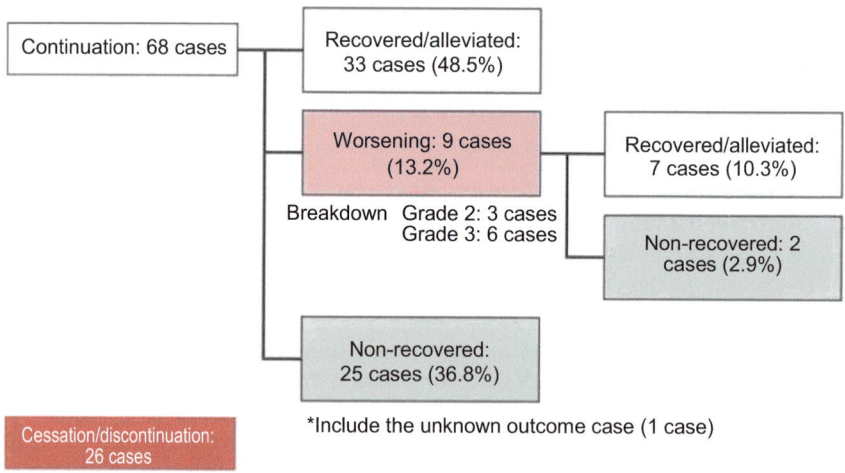

Fig. 4.7 The outcome after continuous administration of everolimus in the appearance of Grade 1 cases of interstitial lung diseases. The final outcome in 68 cases of continuous administration was recovery, alleviation, and non-recovered with after-trouble, and without death. The breakdown in 9 worsened Grade cases of interstitial lung disease after continuous administration was 3 Grade 2 cases (4.4%), 6 Grade 3 cases (8.8%), and no Grades 4 and 5 (fatal) cases. (Cited from Reference [2])

4.2.2.3 Topic

Differentiation from infections: Difficulty in differentiation between infections and drug-induced lung injuries caused by long-term administration of immune suppressors.

Caution must be exercised with mTOR inhibitors as they have immune-suppressing action. mTOR inhibitors were originally used to suppress the immune response after transplants. In long-term administration, patients are susceptible to infections for a long period and differentiation of the infection is thus important. Because frosted glass-like shadows are observed in pneumocystis pneumonia, it is necessary to differentiate it from the frosted glass-like shadows observed in about 30% cases of drug-induced lung injuries (Fig. 4.8 [2]: Chiba Cancer Center).

Temsirolimus-induced lung injuries appeared in 17.38%, and in 0.90% of Grade 5 cases. During the same period, pneumocystis pneumonia occurred in 0.90% of patients and the fatality rate was 0.4% (4 cases). Usually, when a shadow is observed on the images, the case is considered to be a drug-induced lung injury; without any symptoms, the administration is continued and with symptoms, steroids are effective. However, in the case of pneumocystis pneumonia, cases receiving only steroids may become serious, so the differentiation of infections is very important.

Because the KL-6 value with the markers increases for both drug-induced lung injury and pneumocystis pneumonia, β-D glucan, a marker of fungus, is more useful to differentiate the cases. β-D glucan does not increase in the lung injuries induced by mTOR inhibitors but does increase to a high value in pneumocystis pneumonia.

Based on the matters mentioned above, the Interstitial Lung Diseases Study Committee urges consideration of patients' immune condition, especially monitoring of the count of peripheral blood lymphocytes and preventive administration of ST compound drugs according to cases and the differential diagnosis at the appearance.

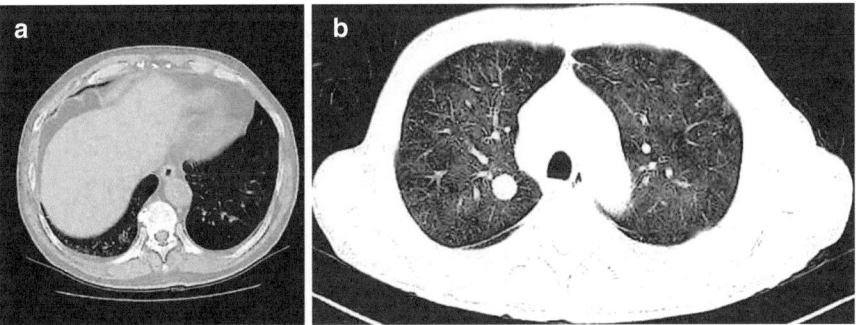

Fig. 4.8 Differentiation from pneumocystis pneumonia (**a**) Lung injury induced by everolimus. (**b**) Pneumocystis pneumonia (Cited from Reference [2])

For this drug, the differential diagnosis is important in the management of toxic events. KL-6, SP-D, and β-D glucan which are usable in Japan have been used for the differentiation.

4.2.2.4 Topic

Toxic events at a high frequency and their influence on subsequent treatment.

Usually, for cases with a history of interstitial pneumonia, anticancer drugs are administered carefully. After drugs with known increased risk of drug-induced lung injury are administered, the subsequent selection of treatment options narrows considerably. For mTOR inhibitors, re-administration after recovery is admitted and the treatment direction in the recovery case is difficult. According to a report by Interstitial Pulmonary Diseases Study Committee, there were 8 cases with a history of drug-induced lung injury before the administration of temsirolimus, and of those, everolimus had been previously administered in 7 of the cases. There were 2 deaths, among which one case was inferred to be active at the administration. As for the decision of administration, after the evidence are taken into consideration, the informed consent will be necessary.

- The drug-induced lung injuries at such frequency may be considered pathologic conditions which are related to the drug efficacy. Even in cases in which a drug-induced lung injury cannot be confirmed, a mild pathologic condition is likely to exist. Various studies have been conducted, and the following reports have been presented. As shown in Fig. 4.9, type II alveolar epithelial hyperplasia, foaming, and retained fat droplets were found in human/mice models. A lot of fat droplets appeared inside the cell cytoplasm in mice alveolar epithelium strains. The manifestation of PPAR-γ was suppressed, and this event was suppressed by administration of PPAR-γ agonist.

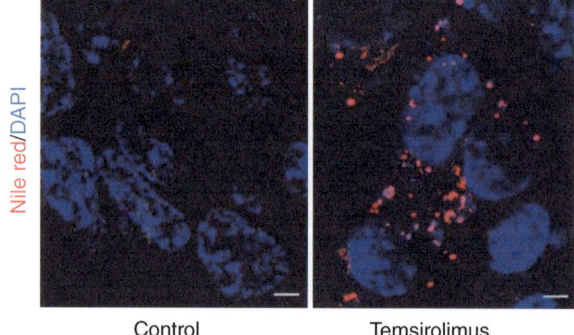

Fig. 4.9 Temsirolimus 20 μM administration for 24 h in MLE12. The fluorescence staining of Nile red (red color) and DAPI (blue color) after temsirolimus (20 μM) at 24 h. The numerous lipid droplets were appeared in the cytoplasm of MLE-12 cells, Scale bars are 5 μm. (Cited from Reference [6])

References

1. Sugiyama S, Sato K, Shibasaki Y, et al. Real-world use of temsirolimus in Japanese patients with unresectable or metastatic renal cell carcinoma: recent consideration based on the results of a post-marketing, all-case surveillance study. Jpn J Clin Oncol. 2020;50:940–7.
2. Afinitor® Tablets 2.5 mg, 5 mg < Radically unresectable or metastatic renal cell cancer > Summary of achievement surveys of specific usage.
3. Gemma A, Kusumoto M, Sakai F, et al. A Study about situation of the appearance of interstitial lung diseases accompanying the use of temsirolimus in treatment of renal cell cancer and risks of the appearance. The 54th Annual Meeting of Japan Society of Clinical Oncology.
4. Duran I, Siu LL, Oza AM, et al. Characterisation of the lung toxicity of the cell cycle inhibitor temsirolimus. Eur J Cancer. 2006;42:1875–80.
5. Afinitor Tablets. Aggregated results of interstitial lung diseases in specific surveys of usage achievement. 2011.
6. Kokoho N, Terasaki Y, Kunugi S, et al. Analyses of alveolar epithelial injury via lipid-related stress in mammalian target of rapamycin inhibitor-induced lung disease. Lab Investig. 2019;99:853–65.

Chapter 5
Proteasome Inhibitor (Bortezomib)

5.1 Bortezomib (Velcade)

- Indications: Multiple myeloma, mantle cell lymphoma, primary macroglobulinemia, lymphoplasmacytic lymphoma.

Bortezomib (Velcade) was approved for the production and sale on October 20, 2006, and was launched on December 1, 2006. At that time, this drug was placed as a specific medicine for multiple myeloma.

5.1.1 Topic

Progress of using first-in-class drug by personal import.
As for bortezomib, a drug-lag yielded during the time until the drug was approved. Interstitial pneumonia appeared in one of the 34 cases of multiple myeloma in the first and second phase studies in Japan. The drug had been used by subjects personally importing it [1]. As a result, a survey by the Japanese Society of Hematology and the Japanese Society of Clinical Hematology revealed 7 cases of lung disorders among 46 cases of the study subjects and 3 cases for death [2].

5.1.1.1 Post-Marketing All-Case Survey in Subjects with Multiple Myeloma

Study period: December 2006–November 2007.
  Subjects: Patients with multiple myeloma.
  Number of subjects: 1010 cases.

Observation period: 3 years.
Results: Reference [3].
ILD incidence: 4.5% (45 cases), 3.45% in Grade 3 or more severe.
Fatal cases: 5 cases (0.50%).
Onset time: 14.5 days in the median value (range: 1–83 days), indicating the early appearance.

5.1.1.2 Analyses of the Image Findings in Cases of Lung Injuries by Expert meetings [4]

Number of aggregated cases: Among 3556 cases compiled in specific achievement surveys and self-reports, there were 83 reported cases of lung injuries.

Frequency of lung injuries: 2.33% (83 cases) (3.77% (31 of 823 cases[1]) in statistic results of specific achievement surveys at the same time).

Onset time: Appearing in 71.1% cases within 6 weeks after administration.
Prognosis: 78.3% (65 of 83 cases) recovered/alleviated.

Image patterns: Among 70 cases in which image information was obtained, drug-induced lung injuries in 36 cases,[2] interstitial pneumonia in 23 cases, increased vascular permeability in 7 cases, hypoxemia in 7 cases. Cases of interstitial pneumonia included DAD type in 3 cases, HP (HR) type in 10 cases, and other in 8 cases. In hypoxemia cases, the only finding on the images was insufficiently expanded lungs and no apparent ILD findings were seen.

5.1.2   Findings from the Survey

5.1.2.1   Topic

Presence of drug-induced lung injuries with specific pathologic conditions

- In bortezomib-induced lung injuries, treatment with steroids is effective in many cases.
- As for image findings, specific pathologic conditions such as increased blood permeability, capillary leak syndrome-like cases (Fig. 5.1), and hypoxia without infiltration were reported [3–5], besides findings of general interstitial pneumonia induced by other drugs, such as DAD and HP (hypersensitivity pneumonia).

---

[1] The results from the specific achievement surveys are considered to be close to actual statistic data.

[2] Because hematology specialists tended to exhaustively report cases of lung findings and there were specificity of blood diseases such as a lot of infections, this data is considered to contain many cases which were not drug-induced lung injuries.

Fig. 5.1 Capillary leak syndrome-like lesion. (Reprinted and partially altered from Miyakoshi S. et al. Blood 2006:107:3492–3494)

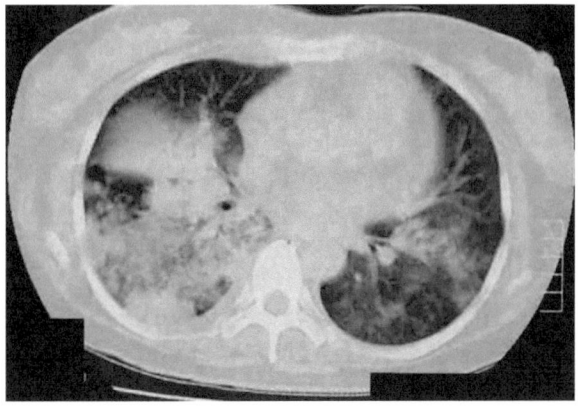

- Capillary leak syndrome-like cases: Those are inferred to be involved by increased permeability pulmonary edema similar to "capillary leak syndrome," which starts with edemas at the vascular walls and just under the bronchial epithelium and progress to pleural effusion and cardiac effusion. The cardiac and circulation dynamics do not show significant variation and it is thus assumed present pathologic conditions and mechanisms are different from those of interstitial pneumonias induced by other drugs. Steroids have been effective for these pathologic conditions.
- Cases expressed as hypoxia without infiltration: Cases which had no abnormal shadow on the images, but hypoxemia occurred.

5.1.2.2 Inside Story

Improvement in usage has been early progressing in cooperation with the Japanese Society of Hematology.

Because drug-induced lung injuries occurred at a high frequency in the users who obtained bortezomib through a personal import, the early handling of the drug was desired. The third-party evaluation committee which was established to investigate the cases summarized specific pathologic conditions associated with bortezomib and reported information on the matter relatively quickly. Simultaneously, the Japanese Society of Hematology compiled questionnaire surveys, and as members of the committee, representative hematologists shared the information. As a result, it was determined that the lung injuries had occurred at a significantly high frequency in cases of hematopoietic stem cell transplantation as pre-treatment and in cases of non-combined steroids at the administration of bortezomib (Velcade). Based on the importance for presence of the transplantation of hematopoietic stem cells and presence or absence of combined steroids, specialists in blood, respiratory organs, and clinical tumors proceeded to study about the management. On February 13, 2007, the midpoint of the survey period, registration of cases of PS 3 and 4 in which deaths and serious cases were notable was prohibited. Because the serious cases varied among facilities, it was suggested to carefully instruct the facilities. This was considered a pioneering handling of facilities' conditions and physicians' conditions.

Finally, the fatality rate of 0.5% is relatively small among various drug-induced lung injuries. Although various problems occurred at the point when subjects personally imported the drug, the risks have been less with early management preparation. The risk management of this drug is considered to be a case in which, led by the company, the third-party evaluation committee and Japanese Society of Hematology worked together significantly and effectively.

References

1. Miyakoshi S, Kami M, Yuji K, et al. Severe pulmonary complications in Japanese patients after bortezomib treatment for refractory multiple myeloma. Blood. 2006;107:3494.
2. Gotoh A, Ohyashiki K, Oshimi K, et al. Lung injury associated with bortezomib therapy in relapsed/refractory multiple myeloma in Japan: a questionnaire-based report from the "lung injury by bortezomib" joint committee of the Japanese society of hematology and the Japanese society of clinical hematology. Int J Hematol. 2006;84:406–12.
3. Yoshizawa K, Mukai HY, Miyazawa M, et al. Bortezomib therapy-related lung disease in Japanese patients with multiple myeloma: incidence, mortality and clinical characterization. Cancer Sci. 2014;105:195–201.
4. Mukai H, Oyashiki K, Kato T, et al. The appearance of lung injuries associated with treatment of bortezomib in Japanese people. Clin Blood. 2011;52:1859–69.
5. Velcade injection 3 mg. The results of interim aggregation (The aggregated results using 2 cycle data in 500 cases). Janssen Pharmaceutical K.K.

Chapter 6
Immune Checkpoint Inhibitors (Nivolumab, Pembrolizumab, Atezolizumab, and Durvalumab)

6.1 Nivolumab (Opdivo) (Fig. 6.1)

- Human-type anti-human PD-1 monoclonal antibodies.
- Indications: Malignant melanoma, radically unresectable or metastatic renal cell cancer, unresectable advanced/recurrent non-small cell lung cancer, healing-unresectable advanced/recurrent stomach cancer with exacerbation after cancer chemotherapy, unresectable advanced/recurrent malignant pleural mesothelioma with exacerbation after cancer chemotherapy, recurrent or refractory classic Hodgkin's lymphoma, recurrent or remote metastatic head and neck cancers, radically unresectable advanced/recurrent esophageal cancer with exacerbation after cancer chemotherapy, healing-unresectable advanced/recurrent MSI-High colon cancer with exacerbation after cancer chemotherapy, and healing-unresectable advanced/recurrent MSI-high rectal cancer with exacerbation after cancer chemotherapy.

6.1.1 All-Case Survey in Subjects with Non-small Cell Lung Cancer

Study period: December 2015–October 2020.
  Subjects: Patients with non-small cell lung cancer.
  Number of subjects: 3612 cases (3606 cases for safety analysis).
  Observation period: 12 months.
  Results: References [2–6], and.
  ILD incidence: 9.57% (345 cases), 3.05% (110 cases) in Grades 3 and 4, and 0.94% (34 cases) in Grade 5.

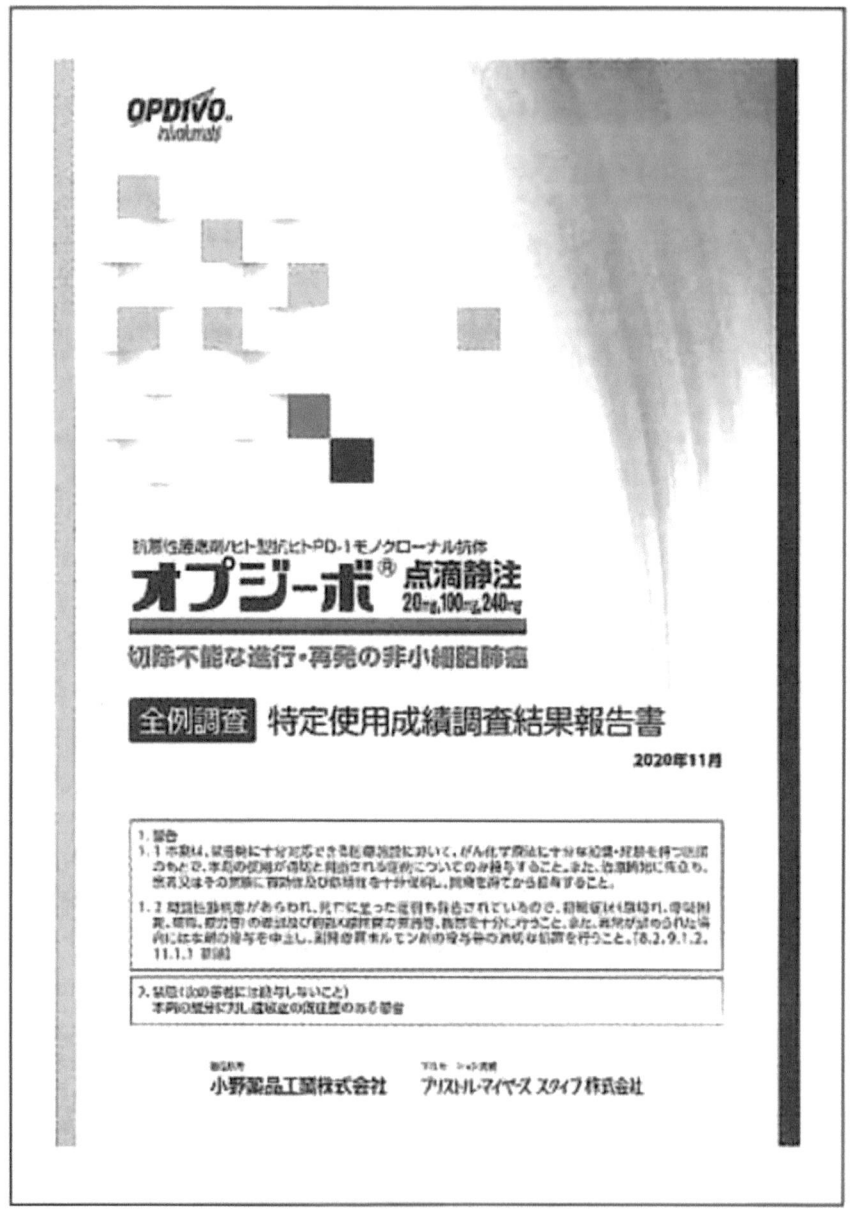

Fig. 6.1 Opdivo® drip infusion 20 mg, 100 mg, 240 mg. A report on the results of specific surveys of usage achievement in unresectable advanced/recurrent non-small cell lung cancers. (Cited from Reference [1])

6.1 Nivolumab (Opdivo)

Mortality in cases with ILD: 9.99%.

Risk factors: Abnormal CT findings, smoking history, and abnormal findings besides lung cancer in the chest CT.

Risk factors involved in fatal cases: ILD patterns and CRP high value as risk factors [5].

Prognosis-updated multivariate analysis (for death): 37 cases of Grade 5 among 238 ILD cases which were evaluated by the expert committee, ILD pattern (DAD), period from the initiation of the administration up to the occurrence (within 60 days), distribution of pleural effusion before the treatment (contralateral or bilateral), CRP change [6].

6.1.2 Findings from the Surveys

6.1.2.1 Topic

Characteristic interstitial pneumonia with immune checkpoint inhibitors.

In many cases, ILD occurs within 2 months after initiation of the administration. In cases where ILD appears within 2 months, the mortality rate is high (Fig. 6.2) [4], which was thus listed as a prognostic factor in the subsequent multivariate analysis [5].

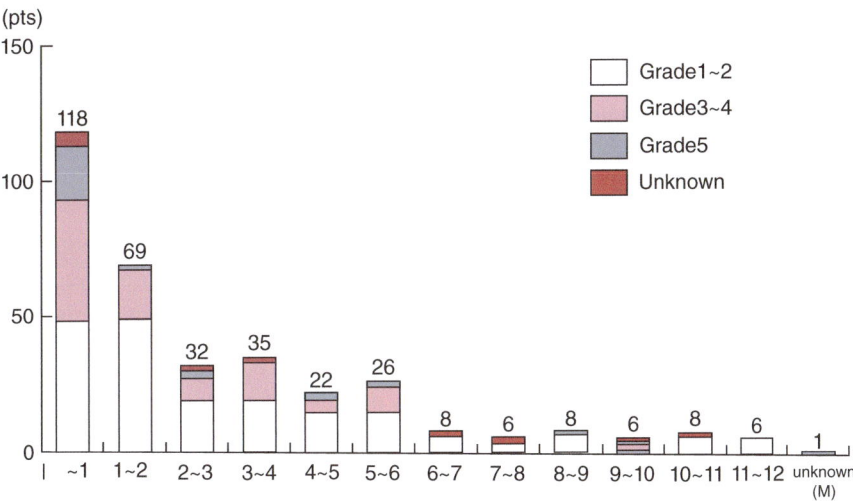

When the same event occurred in the same case, the first event was used.
※Excluding cases of unknown timing

Fig. 6.2 Onset time of drug-induced lung injuries and grade (Cited from Reference [4])

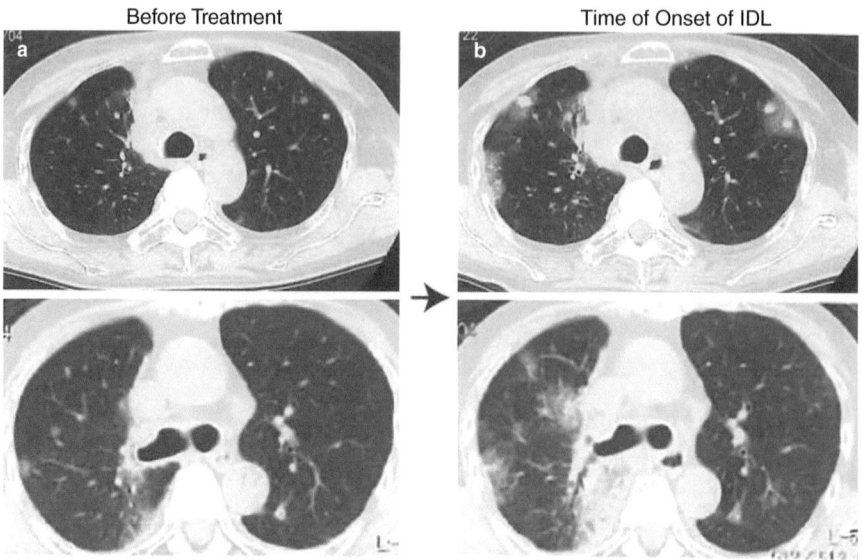

Fig. 6.3 Peritumoral infiltration (PTI). (**a**) Before Treatment. (**b**) Time of onset of ILD

A feature of ILD induced by nivolumab is a population of the cases with specific image pattern. Among 617 ILD cases in the all-case survey, the 155 cases in which the lung CT images were analyzed included 101 cases of interstitial pneumonia with the same pattern as that of ordinary drug-induced interstitial pneumonia and 54 cases with a pattern specific for immune checkpoint inhibitors [6]. Among 54 cases, 24 cases show shadows around the tumors (Fig. 6.3), and other cases were classified into four patterns: a pattern with exacerbation of infections (Fig. 6.4), a pattern with exacerbation of radiation pneumonitis, a pattern with exacerbation of radiation pneumonitis localized in one side on the ipsilateral side, and a pattern with exacerbation of pneumonitis localized ipsilateral to the tumor.

Among those cases, the typical pattern is one with shadows around the tumors. This pattern was found in 27 of 238 cases (11.3%) which were finally analyzed [5]. Since the immune checkpoint inhibitors activate the immune system, we may observe the drug efficacy of aggregated immunocytes around the tumors. Pseudo-progression should be considered in the evaluation of the effect of the immune checkpoint inhibitors. This is a phenomenon that even if the condition is observed as getting worse, subsequently, the effect appears. It is considered difficult to differentiate the ILD specific for the immune checkpoint inhibitors from cases of pseudo-progression.

Figure 6.4 shows a case of worsened infection, which is inferred to lead to the exacerbation of pneumocystis pneumonia. Because pneumocystis pneumonia with high vital reactions is thought to expand the pathologic conditions over the whole lung field, this drug which activates immunity is assumed to aggravate the pathologic conditions.

6.1 Nivolumab (Opdivo)

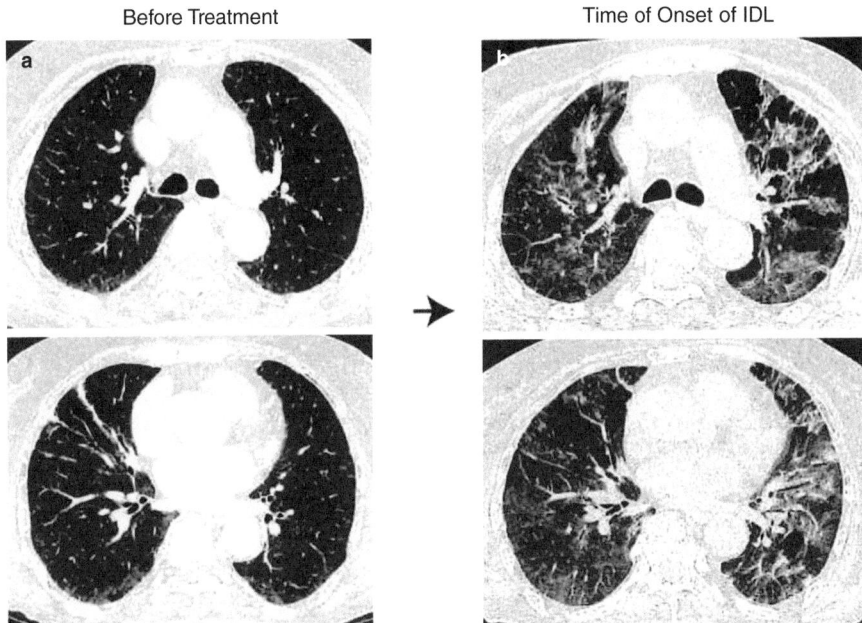

Fig. 6.4 Patterns like intensified infections (pneumocystis pneumonia) (**a**) Before treatment. (**b**) Time of onset of ILD (the night of the day of the first dose) (β-D-glucan: 157 pg/mL). Melanoma patient outcome: Death. (Cited from Reference [6])

Risk factors for the occurrence of drug-induced lung injuries were listed to be abnormal CT findings, smoking history, and abnormal findings besides lung cancer in the chest CT. However, the prevention of any occurrences is not necessarily desired, the risk factors in the fatal cases must be considered as an important matter. In case of immune checkpoint inhibitors, the frequency of ILD case is about 10%. From the final multivariate analysis of the fatal cases, risk factors were ILD pattern, the period from initiation of the administration up to the occurrence, distribution of pleural effusion before the treatment, and high CRP value [5].

Although the features of immune checkpoint inhibitors have been reported as above, the difference among the organs must also be considered. The report values of ILDs around tumors are from the post-marketing all-case survey in the subjects with lung cancer, and it is estimated that the frequency will be less in cases of other types of cancer.

The frequency of the appearance of pneumonitis in different cancer types detected by the anti-PD-1 antibody differs among the organs (Fig. 6.5) [7]. For instance, the frequency is low in the case of melanoma, whereas it is similar between lung cancer and renal cancer. It is unknown why the frequency in renal cancer is close to that in lung cancer.

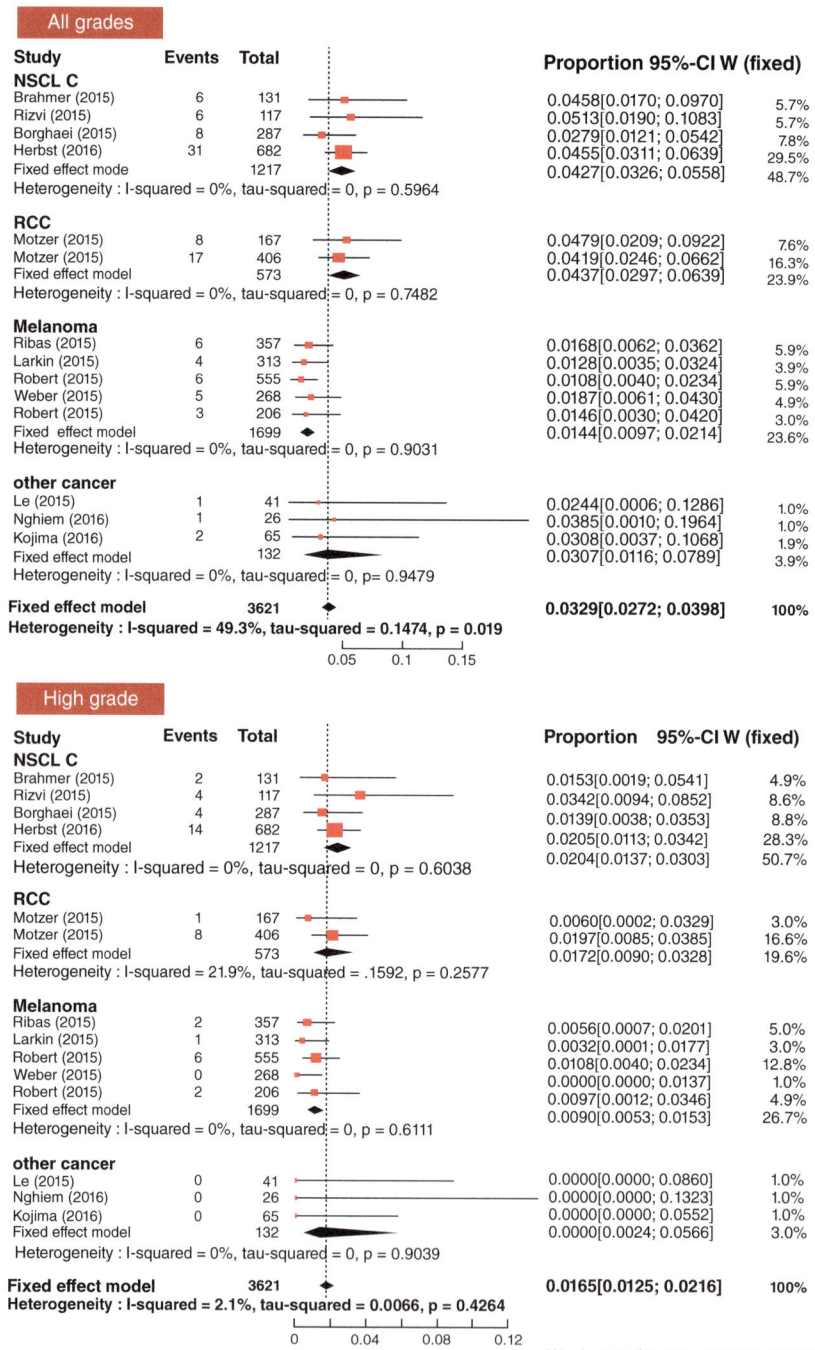

Fig. 6.5 Frequency of pneumonitis in different cancer types by anti-PD-1 antibody (in different grades). (Cited from Reference [7])

A 70 years old female with lung adenocarcinoma. Ground glass opacity surrounding tumors appeared after nivolumab treatment. This finding is named peritumoral infiltration.

Date of CT imaging before nivolumab treatment: 11 months after the completion of radiotherapy. (Cited from Reference [5])

6.2 Pembrolizumab (Keytruda) (Fig. 6.6)

- Human-type anti-human PD-1 monoclonal antibody.
- Indications: Malignant melanoma, radically unresectable or metastatic renal cell cancer, unresectable advanced/recurrent non-small cell lung cancer, radically unresectable urothelial cancer with exacerbation after cancer chemotherapy, recurrent or refractory classic Hodgkin's lymphoma, advanced/recurrent MSI-high solid cancers with exacerbation after cancer chemotherapy, recurrent or remote metastatic head and neck cancers, radially unresectable advanced/recurrent esophageal squamous cell cancer with being positive for PD-L1, and exacerbation after cancer chemotherapy.

6.2.1 Usage-Achievement Surveys in Subjects with Malignant Melanoma and Non-small Cell Lung Cancer

Study period: December 2016–December 2018 (period of the post-marketing survey: February 2017–August 2017).

The post-marketing all-case survey of pembrolizumab has been conducted, and the final report of the usage achievement including other registered cases is reported [8]. The data is not from only the post-marketing all-case survey and it is thus difficult to conduct a simple comparison with other drugs.

Subjects: Patients with unresectable malignant melanoma, unresectable advanced/recurrent non-small cell lung cancer with positive for PD-L1.

Number of subjects: 2805 cases (2739 cases for safety analysis) [7].

Observation period: 1 year.

Results: Reference [7].

ILD incidence[1]: 12.2% (335 cases), 3.94% (108 cases) in Grades 3 and 4, and 1.3% (35 cases) in Grade 5.

Mortality in ILD cases: 10.4%.

---

[1] Because cases of malignant melanoma and other registered cases are included, it cannot be compared simply with Nivolumab (Opdivo).

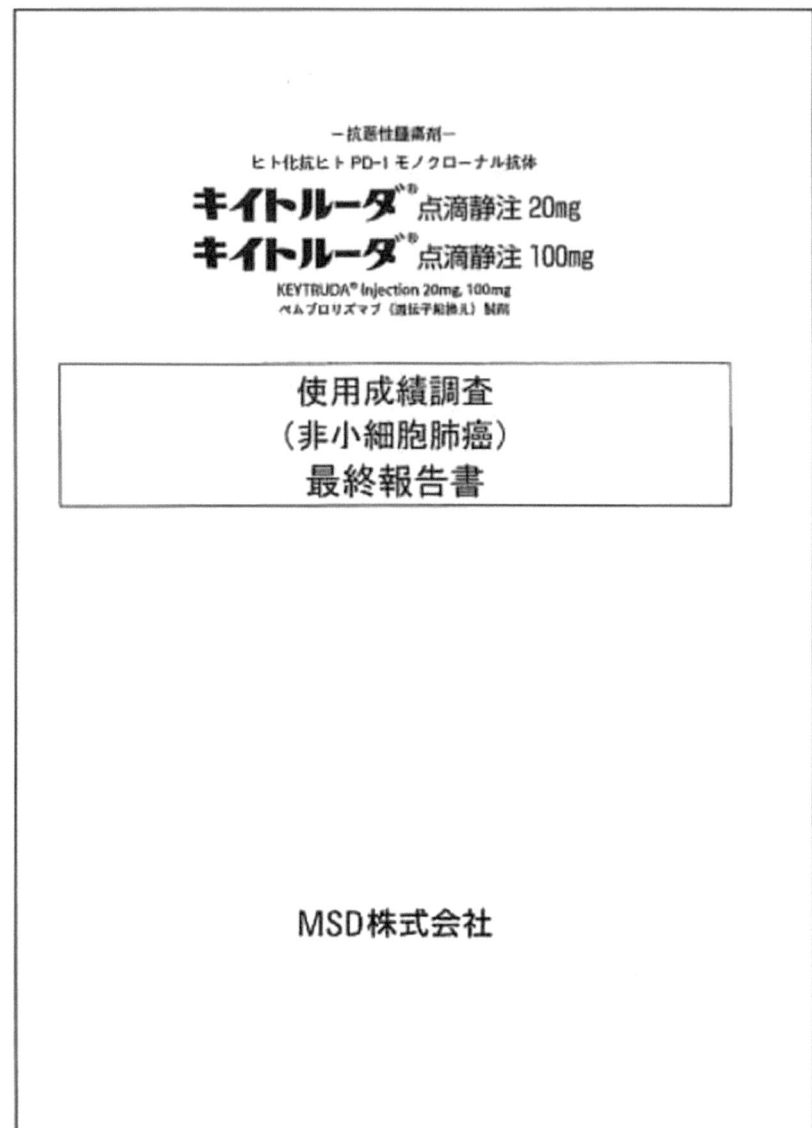

Fig. 6.6 Keytruda® drip infusion 20 mg, 100 mg. A final report on the usage achievement surveys (in non-small cell lung cancer). (Cited from Reference [8])

Risk factors: Hospitalization and outpatient status before initiation of the administration, smoking history, complication in or the medical history of interstitial pneumonia or the respiratory organs/thoracic and mediastinum disorder (Table 6.1).

Risk factors involved in fatal cases: Poor PS, pleural metastasis, LDH 250 IU/L or higher [8].

6.2 Pembrolizumab (Keytruda)

Table 6.1 Multivariate analysis about the side effect of pembrolizumab on the onset of interstitial pneumonia

	n = 2543	% of ILD (events)	Odds ratio (95% CI)
Hospitalization and outpatient before initiation of the administration	Inpatient (n = 1977) Outpatient (n = 566)	13.3% (263) 8.1% (46)	1.76 (1.26–2.44)
Smoking history (ongoing + in the past)	Presence (n = 2098) Absence (n = 445)	13.3% (279) 6.7% (30)	1.97 (1.33–2.93)
Complications: Other	Presence (n = 1416) Absence (n = 1127)	13.9% (197) 9.9% (112)	1.21 (0.92–1.58)
Complications or medical history: Interstitial lung diseases	Present (n = 94) Absence (n = 2449)	22.3% (21) 11.8% (288)	1.87 (1.12–3.11)
Complications or medical history: Respiratory organs, thoracis, and mediastinal disorder SOC (not including special events [a])	Presence (n = 257) Absence (n = 2286)	20.2% (52) 11.2% (257)	1.74 (1.23–2.46)
Complications or medical history: Benign or malignant and details—Unknown neoplasm (including the cysts and polyps) SOC but not including lung cancer	Presence (n = 448) Absence (n = 2095)	15.4% (69) 11.5% (240)	1.27 (0.94–1.71)

[a] Interstitial lung diseases, COPD, asthma are not included

6.2.2 Findings from the Surveys

The fatality rate after the drug-induced lung injuries is about 1% in the nivolumab data, indicating only a little difference. Among 24 fatal cases, the drug-induced lung disorders appeared within 2 weeks after the administration in 13 of 22 cases in which the cases of unknown appearance date are not included [8].

6.3 Atezolizumab (Tecentriq)

- Humanized anti-human PD-L1 monoclonal antibodies.
- Indications: Unresectable hepatic cell cancer, unresectable advanced/recurrent non-small cell cancer, and progressive small cell cancer.

6.3.1 Early Post-Marketing Surveys in Subjects with Non-small Cell Lung Cancer

Study period: April 2018–October 2018.
　Subjects: Patients with non-small cell lung cancer.
　Number of subjects: 2140 of presumed patients administered.
　*Because the numerical value was calculated from cases registered during the period of the early post-marketing surveys, which reported its planned use. The number is not that of the cases reported in the completed submission.
　Results: Reference [8].
　ILD case number: 37 cases.
　Number of deaths in ILD cases: 9 cases.
　Post-marketing all-case survey of atezolizumab (Tecentriq) was conducted, and a report on the midpoint of the survey period was presented.

6.4 Durvalumab (Imfinzi)

- Humanized anti-human PD-L1 monoclonal antibodies.
- Indications: Maintenance therapy after radical chemoradiotherapy in unresectable locally advanced non-small cell lung cancer.

　A post-marketing all-case survey with durvalumab (Imfinzi) has not been conducted.
　Presently, PACIFIC cases in the clinical trial are summarized (Japanese group: immune-mediated harmful events) [3]. An Imfinzi group is a group in which Imfinzi

6.4 Durvalumab (Imfinzi)

was administered after chemoradiation therapy, and a placebo group received only chemotherapy and radiation therapy. As events after the chemotherapy and radiation therapy, pneumonitis occurred in 2 of 40 cases (5%) and 2.5% in Grades 3 and 4. In comparison, pneumonitis in the Imfinzi group was found in 9 of 72 cases (12.5%) and in 1 of 72 cases (1.4%) with Grades 3 and 4. This information indicates that the frequency of pneumonitis in the specific situation is almost similar to the occurrences with other immune checkpoint inhibitors.

Seeing from the overall group, the appearance situation of pneumonitis and radiation pneumonitis is reported to be 161 of 475 cases (33.9%). Including cases of radiation pneumonitis, the frequency in Grade 5 was 5 of 475 cases (1.1%), the frequency with chemotherapy and radiation therapy was 58 of 234 cases (24.8%) and 4 of 234 cases (1.7%) in Grade 5.

In the PACIFIC trial, a study design was applied in which cases of pneumonitis with Grade 2 or more severe were excluded. Although the use of Imfinzi after chemotherapy and radiation therapy is the standard treatment for phase III, Imfinzi may not be administered because of the toxicity after the chemotherapy and radiation therapy. In the future, additional data will be necessary to select cases in which the drug is usable. Because the post-marketing all-case survey of Imfinzi has not yet been completed, it has been difficult to develop the drug usage based on detailed information. Hopefully, the joint study conducted by the company and the Japan Lung Cancer Society will lead to some progress.

6.4.1 Topic

Specificity of the administration of immune checkpoint inhibitors in locally advanced lung cancer.

Imfinzi, regardless of gene mutation, is used as a standard treatment at III phase. Accordingly, among indication cases for the use of immune checkpoint inhibitors, cases having a gene mutation are contained. At the time of recurrence, a molecular-targeted drug may be used with immune checkpoint inhibitors. For example, with nivolumab, because immune checkpoint inhibitors are considered ineffective for cases with a gene mutation, usually a molecular-targeted drug is administered first, and subsequently, an immune checkpoint inhibitor does not become essential. A future problem of treatment with durvalumab in this situation is the possibility that an immune checkpoint inhibitors may be used before a molecular-targeted drug is administered. In a study with osimertinib, the administration of nivolumab is reported to be a risk factor for the occurrence of lung injury. That is, use of a molecular-targeted treatment, especially EGFR-TKI, after immune checkpoint inhibitors may increase the risk for the occurrence of drug-induced lung injury.

A clinical study in which an immune checkpoint inhibitor and a molecular-targeted drug were administered at the same time was commenced, and the results were presented with a highly frequent ILD occurrence. Although no fatal cases occurred, the treatment was discontinued and the clinical study was not completed. In use of EGFR-TKI after use of durvalumab, careful monitoring is required. In addition, the "period after administration of nivolumab and ILD appearance"in a study with osimertinib demonstrate the ILD frequency in the period after administration of nivolumab. ILD frequency decreases in a 5-month interval from after the end of nivolumab administration up to the initial administration of osimertinib. After the end of the administration of immune checkpoint inhibitor, it may be necessary to administer a cytocidal anticancer drug prior to using a molecular-targeted drug.

References

1. Opdivo® drip infusion 20 mg, 100 mg, 240 mg. All-case survey of unresectable advanced/recurrent non-small cell lung cancer. A report on the results of specific surveys of usage achievement.
2. Nakagawa K, et al. Safety profile of nivolumab in patients with NSCLC in Japan: post-marketing all-case surveillance. In: The 59th annual meeting of the Japan Lung Cancer Society; 2018.
3. Kato T, et al. American Society of Clinical Oncology. 2017.
4. Ohe Y, et al. Real-world safety of nivolumab in patients with non-small cell lung cancer (NSCLC) in Japan: interim summary of post-marketing all-case surveillance. Ann Oncol. 2018;29:viii431.
5. Saito Y, et al. Radiographic features and poor prognostic factors of interstitial lung disease with nivolumab for non-small cell lung cancer. Cancer Sci. 2020;112:1495. https://doi.org/10.1111/cas.14710.
6. Baba T, et al. American Thoracic Society. 2017.
7. Wu J, et al. Sci Rep. 2017;7:44173.
8. Keytruda drip infusion 20 mg, 100 mg. A final report on the usage achievement surveys (in non-small cell lung cancer). 2020.

Chapter 7
Neoangiogenesis Inhibitors (Sunitinib, Sorafenib, and Bevacizumab)

As a result of clinical studies, interstitial pneumonia is listed among important toxic events associated with the use of neoangiogenesis inhibitors. This information is included in the package insert. In this section, sunitinib, sorafenib, and bevacizumab, which were investigated in the post-marketing all-case survey are explained.

7.1 Sunitinib (Sutent)

- Kinase inhibitors associated with proliferation of cancer cells.
- Target molecules: VEGFR, PDGFR, and KIT.
- Indications: Imatinib-resistant gastrointestinal stromal tumor, radically unresectable or metastatic renal cell cancer, and pancreatic neuroendocrine cancer.

7.1.1 Post-Marketing All-Case Survey in Subjects with Renal Cell Cancer

Study period: June 2008–December 2008.
  Subjects: Patients with radically unresectable or metastatic renal cell cancer.
  Number of subjects: 664 cases.
  Observation period: June 2008–December 2008, at defined time points.
  Results: Reference [1].
  Incidence of drug-induced lung injury and fatality rate: 0.3% (2 cases), 0.15% (1 case) for the fatality rate.

7.1.2 Findings from the Surveys

As shown above, the frequency of drug-induced lung injuries and mortality with sunitinib are relatively low, at 2/664 cases and 1/664 case, respectively. Thus, drug-induced lung injury is not considered to be a problem influencing the selection of the cases [1].

7.2 Sorafenib (Nexavar)

- Multiple kinase inhibitors associated with proliferation of cancer cells.
- Target molecules: VEGFR, PDGFR, C-Raf, B-Raf, and KIT.
- Indications: Radically unresectable or metastatic renal cell cancer, unresectable hepatic cell cancer, and radically unresectable thyroid cancer.

7.2.1 Post-Marketing All-Case Survey in Subjects with Renal Cell Cancer

Study period: February 2008–September 2009.
Subjects: Patients with renal cell cancer.
Number of subjects: 3255 cases.
Observation period: 12 months.
Results: Reference [2].
Incidence of drug-induced lung injury: 0.15% (5 cases).

7.2.2 Post-Marketing All-Case Survey in Subjects with Renal Cell Cancer/Hepatic Cell Cancer

Study period: April 2008–March 2011.
Number of subjects: 2407 cases of renal cell cancer, 647 cases of hepatic cell cancer.
Results: Reference [3].
Incidence of drug-induced lung injury: 0.33% (8 cases) in renal cell cancer, 0.62% (4 cases) in hepatic cell cancer.
Mortality: 0.17% (4 cases) in renal cell cancer, 0.31% (2 cases) in hepatic cell cancer.
As for the updated information including other reports, refer to the Optimal Clinical Use Guidelines of Nexavar in renal cells (https://pharma-navi.bayer.jp/nexavar/usage-safety/proper-use/guide) [4].

7.2.3 Findings from the Surveys

The frequency of drug-induced lung injury among patients using sorafenib is low.

The frequency of lung injury was higher in patients with hepatic cell cancer than those with renal cell cancer.

In cases of having previous hepatic dysfunction among cases of hepatic cell cancer, toxic events such as hepatic dysfunction are likely to occur and the tendency is present even with a high probability of ILD, and fatality cases are present. In patients with hepatic cell cancer, it is likely that the liver has been already damaged by the virus and is susceptible for hepatic dysfunction. Thus, caution must be exercised.

7.3 Bevacizumab (Avastin) [5]

- Antibody drug (monoclonal antibody) targeting VEGF (vascular endothelial cell proliferation factors) involved in the proliferation of cancer cells.
- Indications: Healing-unresectable advanced/recurrent colorectal cancers, unresectable advanced/recurrent non-small cell lung cancer excluding squamous cell cancer, inoperative or recurrent breast cancer, malignant gliocytoma, ovarian cancer, advanced or recurrent uterocervical cancer, and unresectable hepatic cells.

7.3.1 Post-Marketing All-Case Survey in Subjects with Colon/Rectal Cancers

Study period: June 2007–December 2007.
  Subjects: Patients with colon/rectal cancers.
  Number of subjects: 3727 cases (estimated number of the patients).
  Observation period: 6 months.
  Results: Reference [5].
  Incidence of drug-induced lung injuries/mortality: 0.16% (6 cases)/0.03% (1 case).

7.3.2 Findings from the Surveys

Bevacizumab has been given considerable attention because of a fatal case at an early stage in the clinical developmental step, and focused surveys had thus been conducted. However, the fatal case was only 1/3727 cases, indicating that the frequency is not high.

References

1. Notification on the results of the early post-marketing surveys of Sutent. Pfizer Japan Inc.
2. Akaza H, Oya M, Iijima M, et al. A large-scale prospective registration study of the safety and efficacy of sorafenib tosylate in unresectable or metastatic renal cell carcinoma in Japan: results of over 3200 consecutive cases in post-marketing all-patient surveillance. Jpn J Clin Oncol. 2015;45:953–62.
3. Horiuchi-Yamamoto Y, Gemma A, et al. Drug-induced lung injury associated with sorafenib: analysis of all-patient post-marketing surveillance in Japan. Int J Clin Oncol. 2013;18:743–9.
4. Anon. Optimal clinical use guidelines of Nexavar. Nexavar tablets 200 mg. Osaka: Bayer Yakuhin, Ltd; 2009.
5. Avastin® drip infusion 100 mg/4 mL, 400 mg/16 mL. A report on the aggregated results of side effects in the early post-marketing surveys.

Chapter 8
Other Molecular-Targeted Drugs (Crizotinib, Alectinib, Etc.)

8.1 Crizotinib (Xalkori)

- An ALK inhibitor approved for the first time. Drug-inhibiting signals such as MET, ROS, and ALK.
- Indications: Unresectable advanced/recurrent non-small cell lung cancer positive for the *ALK*-fusion gene or *Ros* mutation.

The drug was used as an ALK inhibitor clinically at its first approval, and since then the indications have been expanded.

8.1.1 Post-Marketing All-Case Survey in Subjects with Non-small Cell Lung Cancer

Study period: 2012–2014.
  Subjects: Patients with unresectable advanced/recurrent non-small cell lung cancer, positive for the ALK-fusion gene.
  Number of subjects: 2120 cases (2028 cases for the safety analysis) [1, 2].
  Observation period: About 1 year.
  Results: References [1, 2].
  ILD incidence: 5.77% (117 cases), 3.45% (70 cases) in Grade 3 or more severe, and 1.13% (23 cases) in Grade 5.
  Mortality: 23.5% (32 cases).
  Onset time: Appeared in 59.0% (69 cases) within 6 weeks.
  Fatality cases: Occurred at a relatively early stage after use of the drug in many cases (Fig. 8.1).

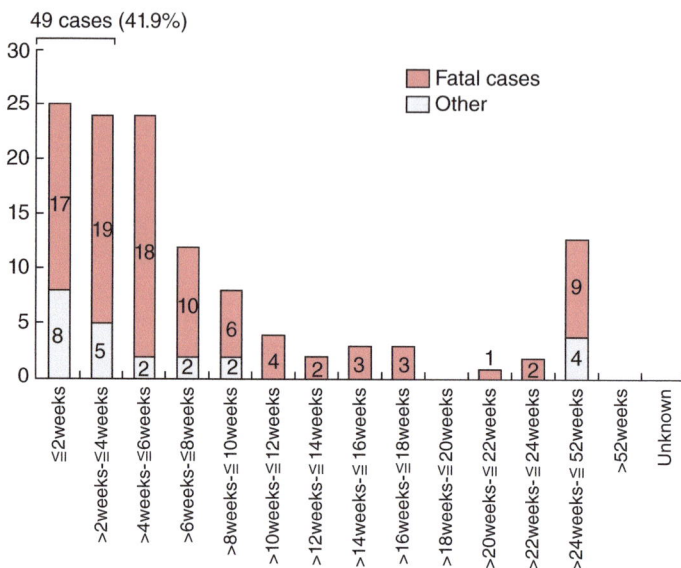

Fig. 8.1 Onset time of drug-induced lung injury: Gray line: Fatal cases, Red line: Others (Reprinted from Reference [2])

Image pattern: DAD appeared in 23.5% (32 cases), pulmonary edema-like shadow was found in 6.9% (8 cases) (typical cases shown in Fig. 8.2d).

Risk factors: Elderly person, poor systemic condition (PS 2–4), smoking history, history of ILD, and presence of pleural effusion.

8.1.2 Findings from the Surveys

The findings of the ILD incidence rate, mortality, and early appearance in time were similar to those seen in EGFR inhibitors (Iressa, Tarceva) (Fig. 8.1).

At the beginning, because many ILD cases appeared within 5 days after the administration of crizotinib, an advisory was announced by the company. However, it is inferred that the drug, being the first-in-class drug, was administered in advanced cases due to high anticipation.

Features of crizotinib are explained below.

1. DAD appeared in 23.5% (Fig. 8.2a, b). Pulmonary edema-like shadow was found in 6.9% (Fig. 8.2c). The typical case was with a shadow shown in Fig. 8.2d.
2. Pleural effusion was listed as a risk factor.

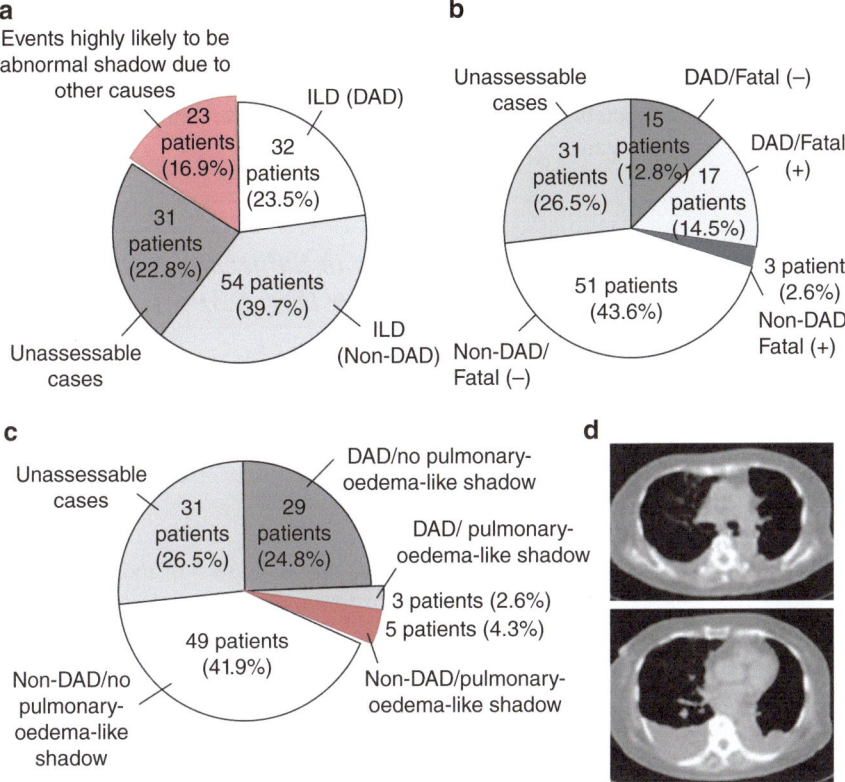

Fig. 8.2 Incidences of ILD assessed by the ILD Independent Review Committee. (**a**) ILD related to crizotinib therapy, or due to other causes (N = 140). (**b**) DAD/non-DAD and fatal (+)/non-fatal (−) ratios of ILD related to crizotinib therapy (n = 117). (**c**) DAD/non-DAD and presence/absence of pulmonary edema-like shadow in the ILD related to crizotinib therapy (n = 117). (**d**) Typical example of pulmonary edema-like shadow. ILD, interstitial lung disease; DAD, diffuse alveolar damage. (Reprinted from Reference [2])

8.1.2.1 Inside Story

The background for making pleural effusion a risk factor—Correspondence by the company, Gemma et al. [2], and medical workers [1, 2].

When the analysis of the results from the post-marketing all-case survey took place, some cases of pleural effusion were noted which were undeniable that they are related to the drug. All cases of pleural effusion which continued during the course of treatment were re-investigated. As the result, a certain number of cases with pulmonary edema-like shadow were detected and the relatively early death cases were also found. From those findings, the cases were suspected to be the drug-induced and a warning for the matter had been raised. The analysis finally led to listing pleural effusion as a risk factor for drug-induced lung injury.

8.2 Alectinib (Alecensa) [3, 4]

- The drug inhibits ALK and RET, approved as an ALK inhibitor.
- Indications: Unresectable advanced/recurrent non-small cell lung cancer positive for the ALK-fusion gene.

8.2.1 Post-Marketing All-Case Survey in Subjects with Non-small Cell Lung Cancer (Fig. 8.3)

Study period: September 2014–March 2017.

Subjects: Patients with unresectable advanced/recurrent non-small cell lung cancer positive for the ALK-fusion gene.

Number of subjects: 1251 cases (1221 cases for the safety analysis).

Observation period: 18 months.

Results: References [3, 4].

ILD incidence: 3.87% (47 cases), 0.73% (9 cases) in Grade 3 or more severe.

Fatal cases: One case (a study by the expert committee: One of 25 cases of ILD).

Onset time: Within 8 weeks after the administration (33%).

Image pattern: 3 DAD cases (12%) among 25 cases investigated in the ILD advisers meeting [4], 7 cases of COP/CEP-like patterns (28%), 11 cases of faint infiltration or acute HP-like patterns (44%) (Table 8.1, Fig. 8.4). Even such cases of traction bronchiectasis or volume reduction showed alleviation (Fig. 8.5). A pneumonedema-like pattern was detected only in one case.

8.2.2 Findings from the Surveys

The ILD incidence cannot be said to be lower than that with crizotinib, but the mortality is low in high grades.

The onset time was different from that seen with crizotinib, which appeared mainly at an early stage after administration.

The DAD incidence was 12%, lower than those with EGFR-TKI or crizotinib (one third to one fourth) [4].

The image pattern is different from that of crizotinib.

As for factors of different pathologic conditions of drug-induced lung injuries with those seen with crizotinib, an ALK inhibitor, it is presumed that the inhibition signal spectrum includes other routes such as ROS or RET inhibition, differs between both drugs and other ingredients of the drugs make an influence. It is still unknown whether the appearance of pulmonary edema-like findings results from the ALK inhibitor.

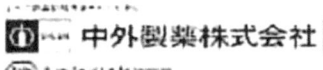

Fig. 8.3 Surveys of usage achievement of Alecensa® capsule. Final report. (Cited from Reference [5])

Table 8.1 CT image patterns at the onset of alectinib-induced ILD

Image patterns	Number of cases (%)
AIP-like pattern	3 cases (12%)
COP/CEP-like pattern	7 cases (28%)
Faint infiltration or acute HP-like pattern	11 cases (44%)
NSIP 1 like pattern	1 case (4%)
GGA + thickened image of inter-lobular interval + infiltrative shadow	1 case (4%)
Pneumonedema-like pattern	1 case (4%)
Indeterminable	1 case (4%)
Total number of cases	25 cases

(Cited from Reference [4])

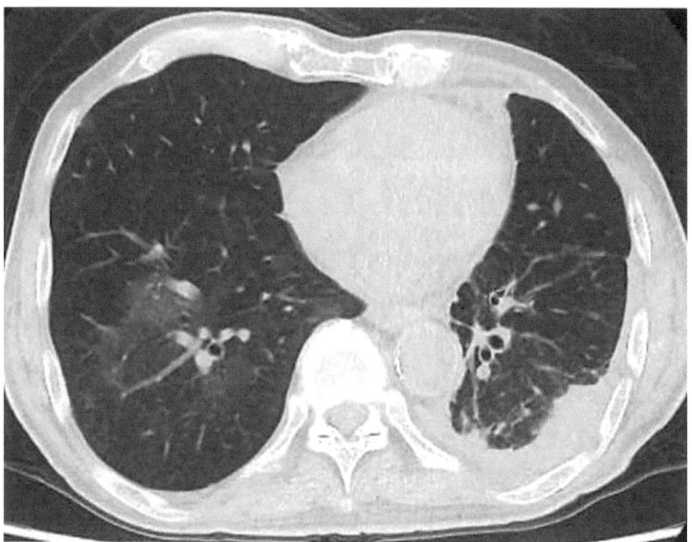

Fig. 8.4 ILD at the administration of alectinib. (Cited from Reference [4])

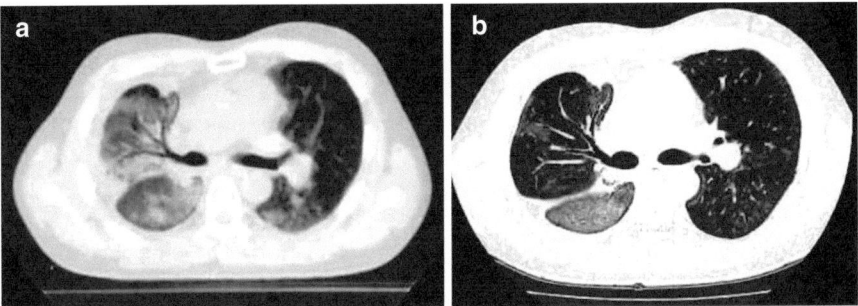

Fig. 8.5 ILD at the administration of alectinib. (**a**) Appearance of lung injury in both lungs, found reduced volume in the right superior lobe. (**b**) Recovery after treatment with steroid pulse (Cited from Reference [4])

8.3 Trastuzumab (Herceptin)

- Anti-HER2 humanized monoclonal antibody.
- Indications: Breast cancer with the appearance of excessive HER2, healing-unresectable advanced/recurrent gastric cancer.

In achievement surveys in Japan and special surveys of subjects with metastatic breast cancer, severe interstitial lung diseases appeared in 7 of 1123 cases for the safety analysis (0.5%) [6] (Fig. 8.6). The incidence of interstitial lung diseases with this drug is considered to be relatively low.

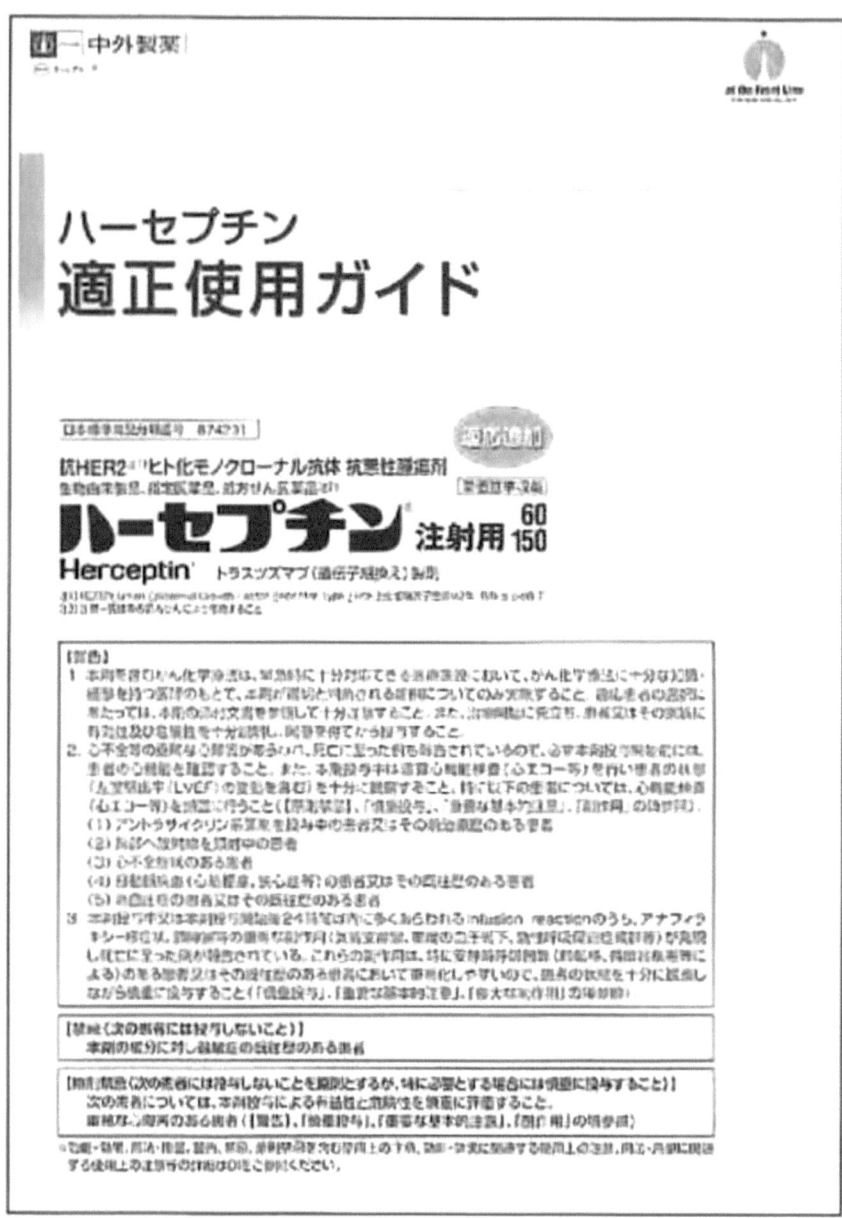

Fig. 8.6 Optimal Clinical Use Guidelines of Herceptin. (Cited from Reference [6])

8.4 Pertuzumab (Perjeta)

- Humanized monoclonal antibody to the domain with a dimer formation in a region outside human HER2 cells.
- Indications: Breast cancer positive for HER2.

8.4 Pertuzumab (Perjeta)

ILD in 9 of 407 cases is reported in CLEOPATRA study in subjects with HER2 positive metastatic/recurrent breast cancer [7] (Fig. 8.7). In achievement surveys with 277 cases registered from October 2013 to September 2015, ILD was found in 1 of 261 cases for the safety analysis [8] (Fig. 8.8). The incidence of ILD with this drug is considered to be relatively low.

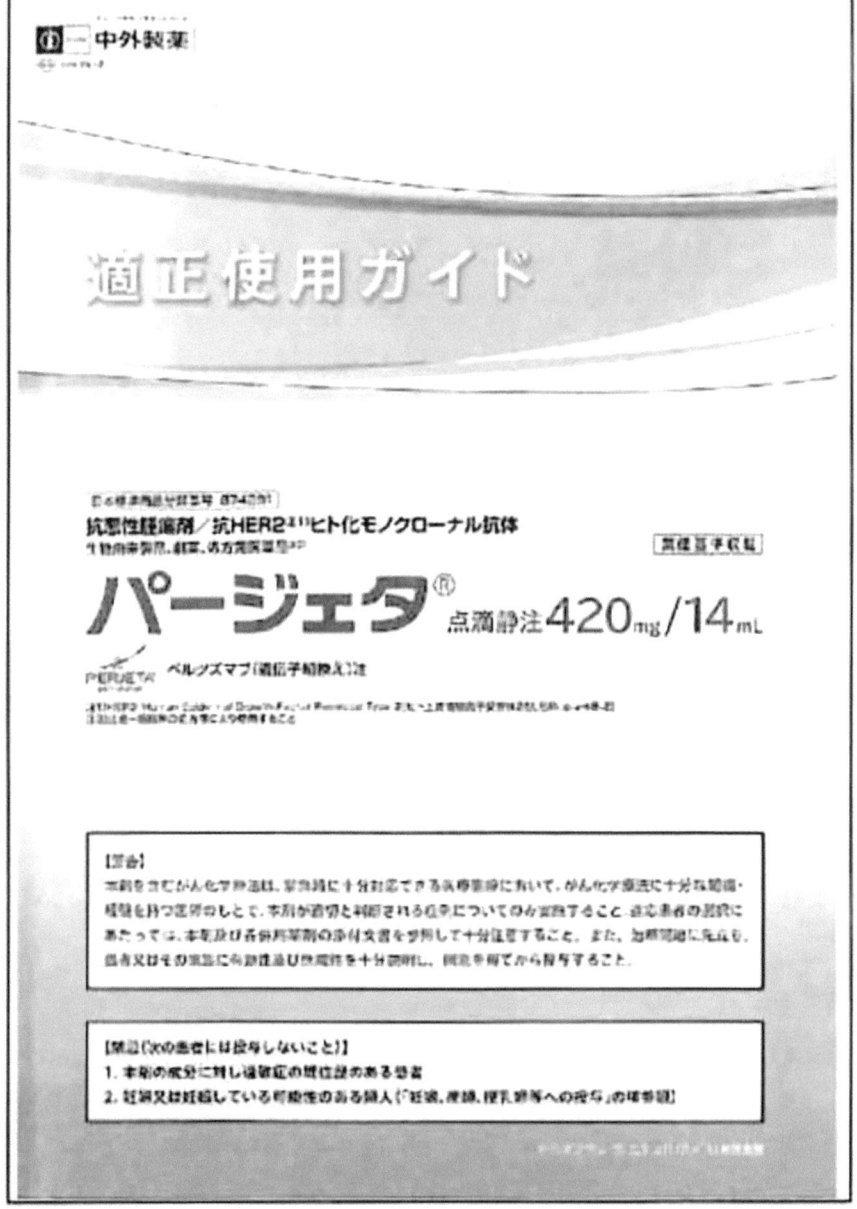

Fig. 8.7 Optimal clinical use guidelines of Perjeta drip infusion 420 mg/14 mL. (Cited from Reference [7])

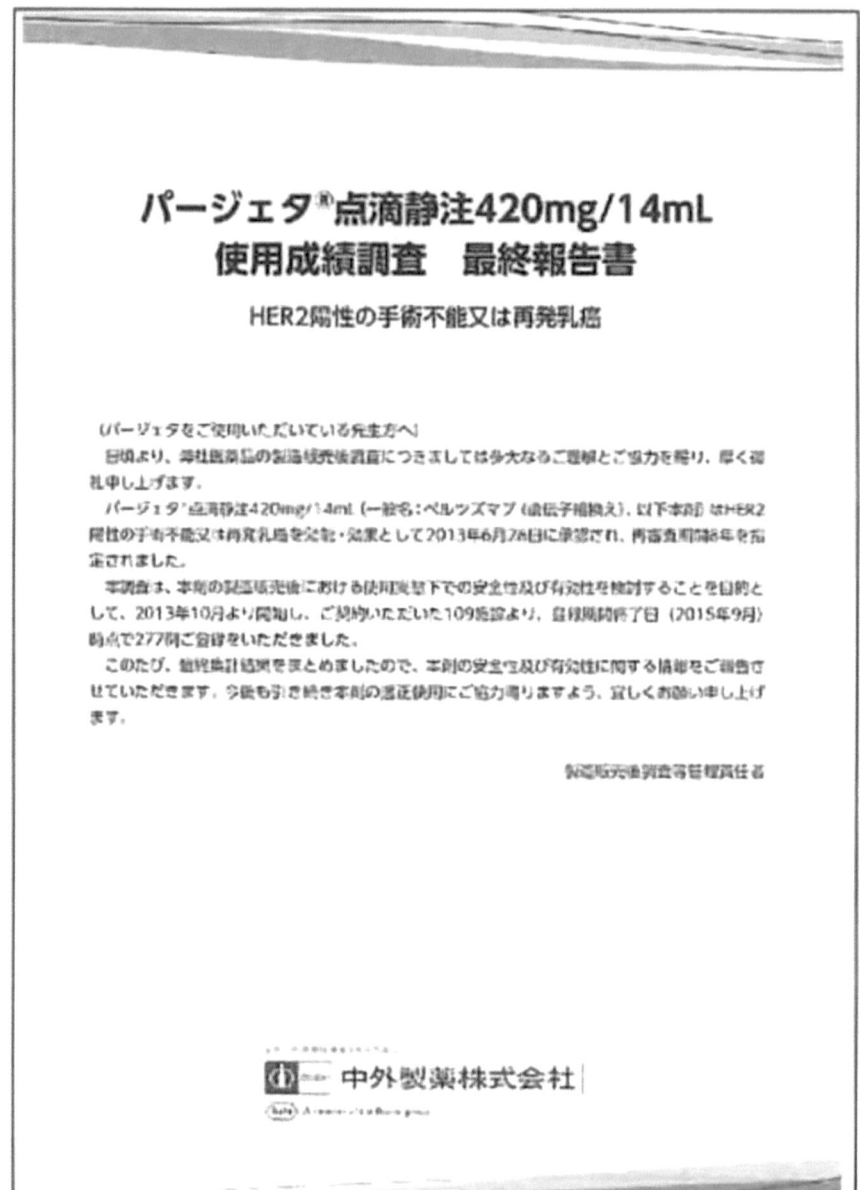

Fig. 8.8 Surveys of use achievement of Perjeta drip infusion 420 mg/14 mL. Final report. (Cited from Reference [8])

8.5 Palbociclib (Ibrance)

- CDK4/6 inhibitor.
- Indications: Hormone receptor positive and HER2 negative inoperable or recurrent breast cancer.

Drug-induced lung injuries appeared in 4 of 444 cases (0.9%) and 3 of 345 cases (0.9%) with this drug, similar to placebo (0.9%, 1.2%) in international joint phase III studies (PALO-MA-2, PALOMA-3). Among patients to whom palbociclib was administered in Japan from September 2017 to December 2019, there were 56 events related to interstitial lung diseases and 4 fatal cases (Table 8.2). Attention to future information is necessary.

Table 8.2 Post-marketing appearance situation

Side effects (PT)	Severe		Non-severe	No information	Total
	Other than death	Death			
Interstitial lung diseases	18 cases	3 cases	19 cases	11 cases	51 cases
Pulmonary disorders	–	1 case	–	–	1 case
Pneumonitis	3 cases	–	–	–	3 cases
Radiation pneumonitis	–	–	–	1 case	1 case
Total	21 cases	4 cases	19 cases	12 cases	56 cases

Events included in interstitial lung disease (narrow-range + wide-range) of MedDRA AMQ and basic words "lung injury" of MedDRA were aggregated

Information on January 24, 2020, in cases whose initial information were obtained during a period from September 27, 2017 to December 31, 2019 (cited from Reference [9])

References

1. Ueno N, Banno S, Endo Y, et al. Treatment status and safety of crizotinib in 2028 Japanese patients with ALK-positive NSCLC in clinical settings. Jpn J Clin Oncol. 2019;49:676–86.
2. Gemma A, Kusumoto M, Kurihara Y, et al. Interstitial lung disease onset and its risk factors in Japanese patients with ALK-positive NSCLC after treatment with Crizotinib. J Thorac Oncol. 2019;14:672–82.
3. Masuda N, Ohe Y, Gemma A, et al. Safety and effectiveness of alectinib in a real-world surveillance study in patients with ALK-positive non-small-cell lung cancer in Japan. Cancer Sci. 2019;110:1401–7.
4. Kusumoto M, Masuda N, Ohe Y, et al. Safety study in achievement surveys of specific usage of alectinib for ALK-positive non-small cell lung cancer—especially, as for interstitial lung disease. The Annual Meeting of the Japan Lung Cancer Society in 2018.
5. Achievement surveys of usage of Alecensa® capsule. Final report.
6. Optimal Clinical Use Guidelines of Herceptin. Revised edition in March, 2008.
7. Optimal Clinical Use Guidelines of Perjeta drip infusion 420 mg/14 mL, Revised edition in October 2018.
8. Achievement surveys of use of Perjeta drip infusion 420 mg/14 mL. Final report. 2018.
9. Requested matters to medical workers: Notable side effects of Ibrance capsules and tablets and countermeasures.

Chapter 9
Antibody-Drug Conjugates (ADC) (Trastuzumab Emtansine and Trastuzumab Deruxtecan)

9.1 Trastuzumab Emtansine (T-DM1, Kadcyla) [1, 2]

- An antibody-drug conjugate (ADC) in which trastuzumab and DM1 (derivative of maytansine) having the polymerization inhibiting action of tubulin is combined by linker.
- Indications: HER2 positive inoperable or recurrent breast cancer.

Interstitial lung diseases were found in 7 of 490 cases (1.4%) in an international phase III study in subjects with inoperable or recurrent breast cancer and in 1 of 73 cases (1.4%) in a phase II study in Japan [1] (Fig. 9.1). An analysis (KATHERINE study) on the use of trastuzumab emtansine in postoperative adjuvant chemotherapy showed 21 cases (2.8%) of interstitial lung disease in 740 subjects, and the 11 cases were radiation pneumonitis [2] (Fig. 9.2). In addition, it was reported that all 21 cases received radiation therapy. Compared to other ADCs, the frequency of drug-induced lung injuries was lower.

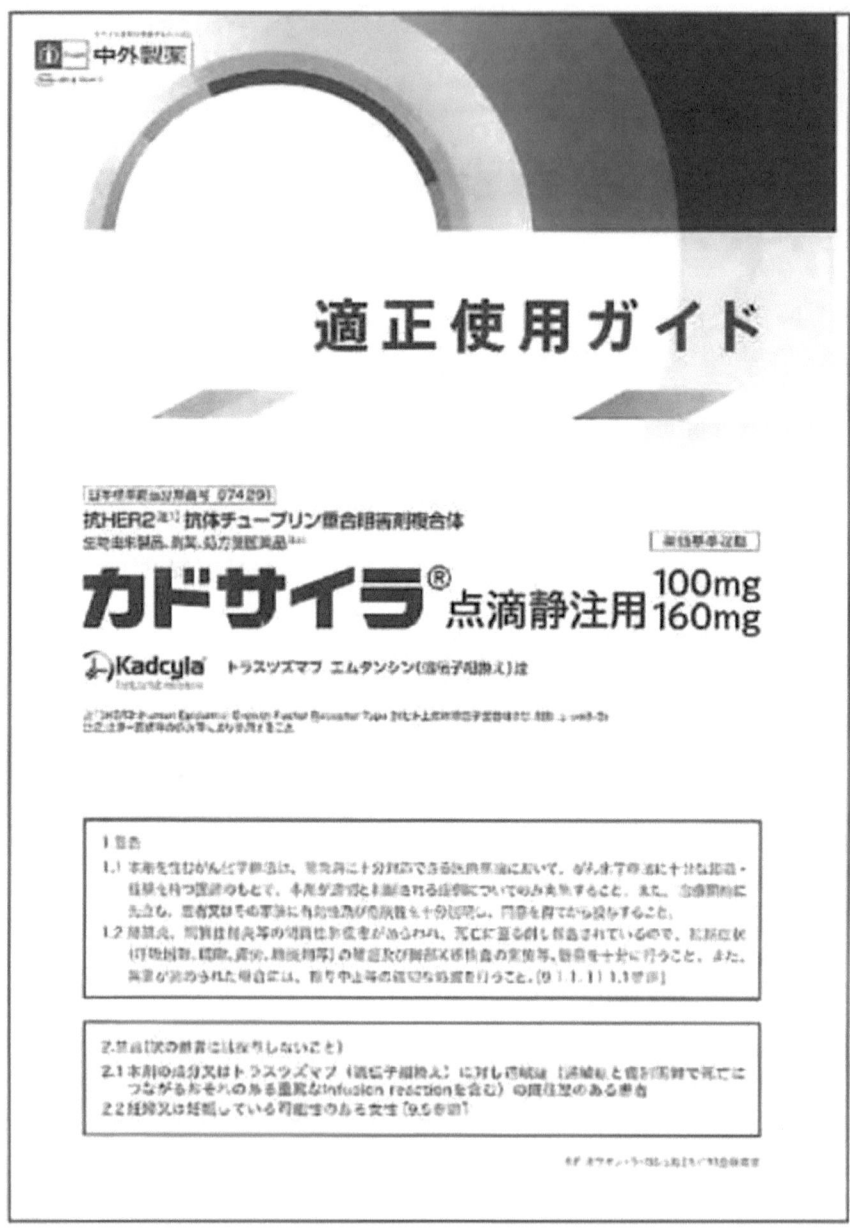

Fig. 9.1 Optimal clinical use guidelines of Kadcyla drip infusion 100 mg and 160 mg. (Cited from Reference [1])

9.1 Trastuzumab Emtansine (T-DM1, Kadcyla)

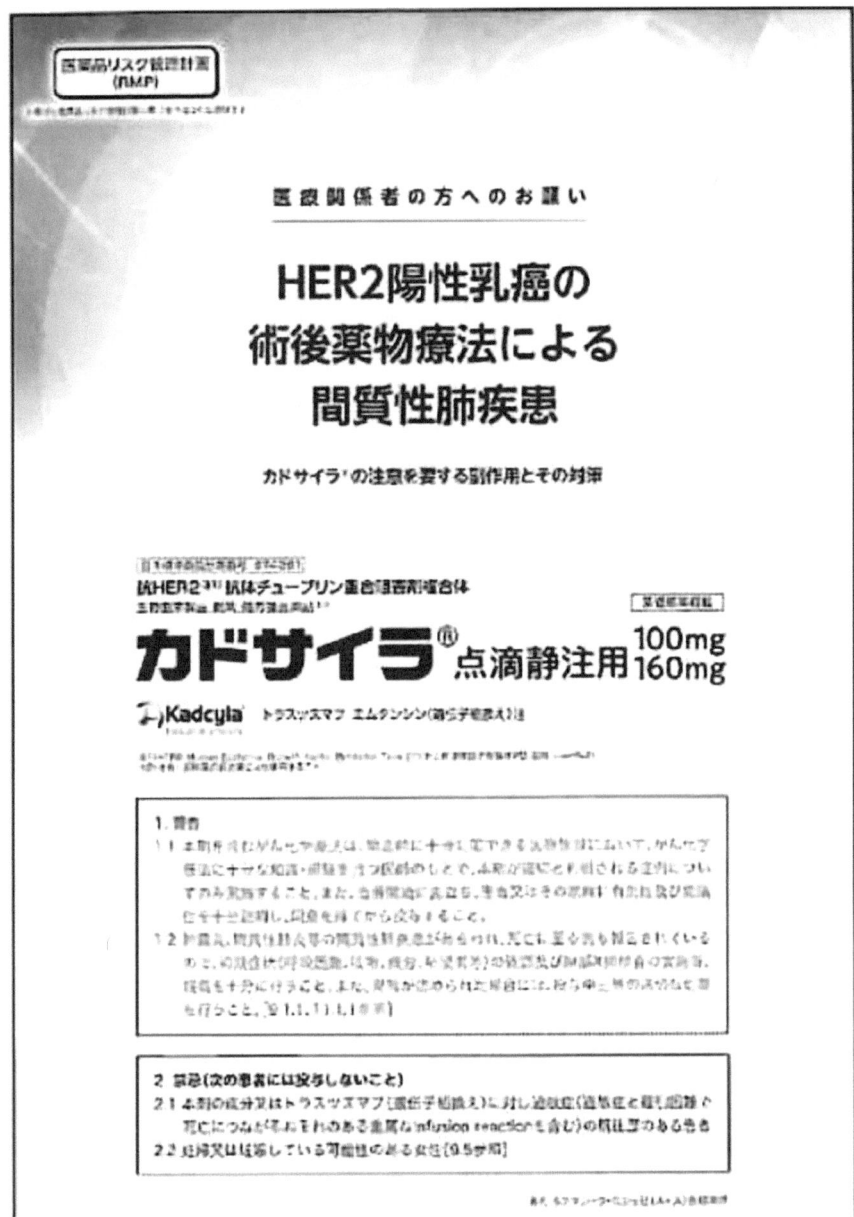

Fig. 9.2 Kadcyla drip infusion 100 mg and 160 mg. Interstitial lung diseases induced by postoperative drug therapy for HER2 positive breast cancer. (Cited from Reference [2])

9.2 Trastuzumab Deruxtecan (Enhertu) (Fig. 9.3) [3]

- An antibody-drug conjugate (ADC) in which an antibody targeting human epithelial proliferative factors-receptor 2 (HER2) and a drug having topoisomerase I inhibiting action are combined.

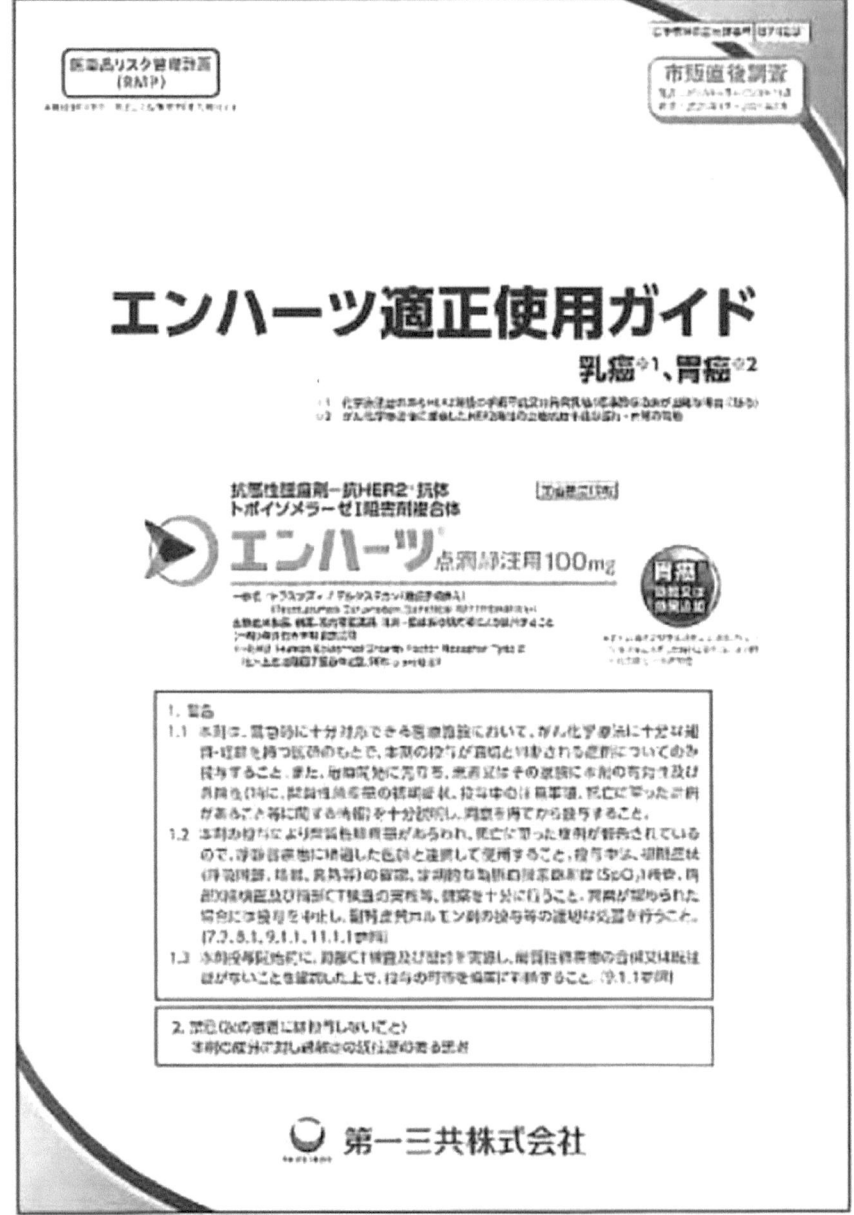

Fig. 9.3 Optimal clinical use guidelines of Enhertu. (Cited from Reference [3])

9.2 Trastuzumab Deruxtecan (Enhertu)

- Indications: HER2 positive inoperative or recurrent breast cancer with history of chemotherapy (limited to cases that the standard treatment is difficult), HER2-positive healing-unresectable advanced/recurrent gastric cancer worsened after cancer chemotherapy.

A characteristic of this drug is the point that the special linker binding the antibody and the drug is cut by the tumor cells. This technical development of a drug combined with antibodies at a constant rate enables the effects of the drug to be successfully exerted at a much higher degree than that of conventional ones. Since its launch in May 2020, the effects have been recognized.

Conversely, drug-induced lung injuries have been occurring at a certain frequency. As of February 2021, an advisory is on the homepage of PMDA. The results of the post-marketing survey have not been yet reported. The results of the clinical studies are as follows.

9.2.1 Clinical Study (Partially Revised from Reference [3])

9.2.1.1 Study U201

Subjects: Patients with HER2 positive inoperable or recurrent breast cancer, also with a history of T-DM1 treatment at a dose of 5.4 mg/kg.
Number of subjects: 184 cases.

Results

ILD incidence: 8.2% (15 cases) at the time of the approval application for production and sales (data cut-off: March 21, 2019) and 13.6% (25 cases) at the time of the newest data cut-off (August 1, 2019).

ILD incidence in Japanese patients (30 cases): 23.3% (7 cases) at the time of the approval application for production and sales (data cut-off: March 21, 2019) and 30% (9 cases) at the time of the newest data cut-off (August 1, 2019).

Death cases: 1.6% (3 cases) at the time of the approval application for production and sales (data cut-off: March 21, 2019) and 2.2% (4 cases) at the time of the newest data cut-off (August 1, 2019).

Onset time: Day 127 (median value: 35–338 days) after the administration at the time of the newest data cut-off (August 1, 2019).

9.2.1.2 Study J202

Subjects: Patients with HER2-positive progressive gastric adenocarcinoma and those with adenocarcinoma at the gastroesophageal joint region, which became worse after treatment of two regimens with trastuzumab of 6.4 mg/kg, a platinum-containing drug, and antimetabolic drugs.
Number of subjects: 125 cases.

Results

ILD incidence rate: 9.6% (12 cases).
ILD incidence in Japanese patients (99 cases): 11.1%(11 cases).
Onset time: 84.5 days (median value: 36–638 days).

9.2.1.3 Analysis Results of the Initial Doses and Cancer Types

The number of subjects: 645 cases.

Results

ILD incidence and fatality rate: 11.2% (72 cases), 1.6% (10 cases).
ILD incidence and fatality rate in Japanese patients (316 cases): 16.1% (51 cases), 0.6% (2 cases).
Onset time: 153 days (−15–582 days).

9.2.2 Findings from the Surveys

The results of Study U201 in breast cancer found that drug-induced lung injuries occurred in 30% of the Japanese patients, a high rate. The median value of the onset time was 127 days, ranging from 35 to 338 days, which indicates that it may occur at any time.

In Study J202 with gastric cancer, the ILD rate was 9.6% and 11.1% in Japanese patients. The onset time was 84.5 days, ranging from 36 to 638 days. Because of the considerable variability, there is no defined peak time of onset.

In the analyses regardless of initial doses and cancer types, the ILD incidence was 11.2% and the mortality was 1.6%. In Japanese patients, the incidence was 16.1% and the mortality was 0.6%. The incidence was higher in Japanese patients, but the mortality was smaller. In Japanese, usually, drug-induced lung injuries cause DAD, leading to death in many cases. When drug-induced lung injuries occur, while the re-administration becomes possible after recovery if they are Grade 1 cases during the clinical trial, it is presumed that because Japanese physicians managed the cases relatively strictly, the number of the fatal cases were smaller.

In analyses integrating the results of 5 studies, the risk of interstitial lung diseases is high in Japanese patients who received 10 or more regimens of chemotherapy in the past (Table 9.1).

Among lung disorders induced by this drug, infiltration shadows such as an organizing pneumonia (OP) pattern are detected in about 70% cases (Table 9.2 and Fig. 9.4). Many cases may have a concomitant image pattern mainly with grand glass shadows.

9.2 Trastuzumab Deruxtecan (Enhertu)

Table 9.1 ILD risk factors of the patients regardless of the initial dose and cancer type [1]

Risk factor [2]	Comparison	Odds ratio (95% CI) [3]	p value
Countries of the study	Japan vs other countries	3.1 (1.8, 5.3)	<0.001
Number of regimens of chemotherapy in the past or molecular-targeted treatment	10 or more regimens vs less than 10 regimens	2.4 (1.4, 4.3)	0.002

Table 9.2 The appearance[a] of different image patterns in patients regardless of the initial dose and cancer type[b]

	CTCAE Grade[c]					
Image pattern	1	2	3	4	5	Total
Total	22	34	3	3[d, e, f]	10	72
Diffuse alveolar damage (DAD)	0 (0.0)	2 (5.9)	2 (56.7)	3 (100.0)	9 (90.0)	16 (22.2)
Organizing pneumonia (OP) like type	20 (90.9)	28 (82.4)	1 (33.3)	0 (0.0)	0 (0.0)	50 (69.4)
Hypersensitive pneumonia (HP) like type	2 (9.1)	3 (8.8)	0 (0.0)	0 (0.0)	0 (0.0)	5 (6.9)
Nonspecific interstitial pneumonia (NSIP) like type	0 (0.0)	1 (2.9)	0 (0.0)	0 (0.0)	0 (0.0)	1 (1.4)
Other/unconfirmed	0 (0.0)	0 (0.0)	0 (0.0)	0 (0.0)	0 (0.0)	0 (0.0)

[a] The severity is based on the evaluation by ILD independent evaluation committee
[b] The results of five clinical studies (Study J101, Study U201, Study J102, Study A104, Study A103) ($N = 645$)
[c] The evaluation was based on CTCAE Grade Ver. 5.0
[d] An event of respiratory failure appeared in 1 patient from Study U201, and the patient then died. The severity evaluation of the respiratory failure by the ILD independent evaluation committee at the time of the approval application for production and sales was Grade 4, and subsequently, it was changed to Grade 5 after re-evaluation and the death was evaluated to be caused by ILD
[e] A patient in Study J101 died after the data cut-off. The death was evaluated to be caused by ILD by the ILD independent evaluation committee
[f] A patient in Study J101 died 38 days after final administration of the study drug. The death was evaluated to be caused by ILD and the disease progression by the ILD independent evaluation committee

1. The results of five clinical studies (Study J101, Study U201, Study J102, Study A104, Study A103) ($N = 645$).
2. Factors selected in the final model were two factors, including countries of the study and the number of regimens of chemotherapy in the past and molecular-targeted treatment.
3. The odds ratio was calculated after other factors selected were adjusted.

In-company document: Outline of clinical safety: Harmful events (Approved on March 25, 2020. CTD 2.7.4.2). (Cited from Reference [3].

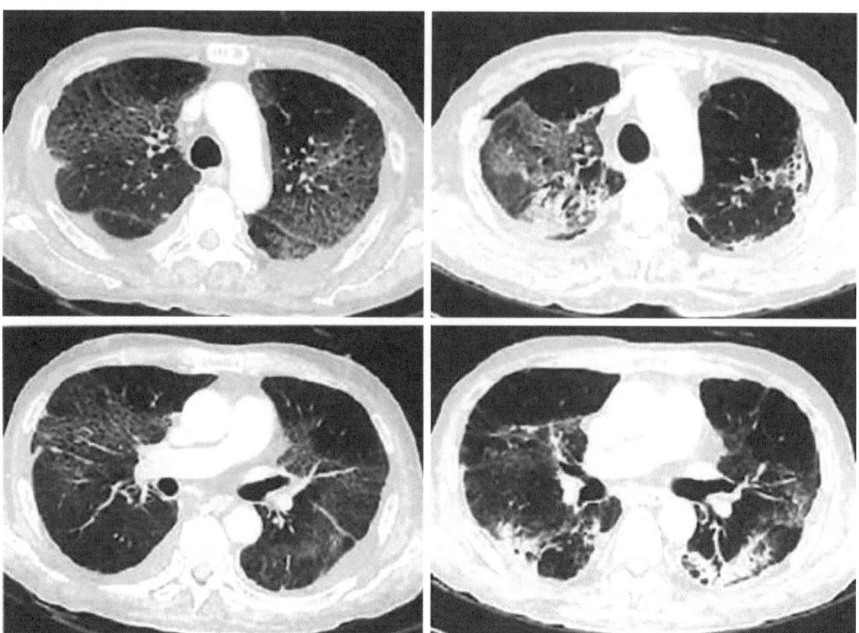

Fig. 9.4 Infiltration shadows (Cited from Reference [3])

In-company document: Additional document for the application. Clinical characteristics of interstitial lung diseases induced by DS-8201a (trastuzumab deruxtecan) and post-marketing safety measures (cited from Reference [3]).

9.2.2.1 Topics

Cautions during COVID-19 epidemic period.

In addition, the image findings of this drug resemble those of COVID-19 that a differential diagnosis is difficult. Although the PMDA and the Japanese Respiratory Society have issued an advisory, its correspondence is required only to facilities where PCR examination is possible. Because the clinical symptoms such as pyrexia, non-productive cough, and shortness of breath seen in drug-induced interstitial pneumonia are also observed in COVID-19, if other symptoms such as impaired taste are absent, a differential diagnosis is difficult. In case that a drug which is assumed to induce drug-induced lung disorders in 30% of cases is administered, during the COVID-19 epidemic, cautions for COVID-19 must be exercised considerably carefully, and clinically, diagnosis will be very difficult. This drug is estimated to be also effective for cases of having the treatment history of 10 regimens or more. Thus, this drug is highly anticipated. In administering the drug to such cases, a system for diagnosis with a PCR must be in place.

References

1. Optimal Clinical Use Guidelines of Kadcyla drip infusion 100 mg and 160 mg. Revised in October 2019.
2. Interstitial lung diseases induced by postoperative drug therapy for HER2 positive breast cancer. Notable side effects of Kadcyla and its countermeasures. 2020.
3. Optimal Clinical Use Guidelines of Enhertu. Daiichi Sankyo Co., Ltd. Revised in December 2020.

Chapter 10
Anticancer Drugs (TS-1, Taxanes, CPT-11, Platinum-Containing Drugs, Etc.)

The risk of drug-induced lung injuries at the clinically trial step is considered to be relatively high with irinotecan hydrochloride, vinorelbine tartrate, gemcitabine hydrochloride, and amrubicin hydrochloride (Table 10.1). The number of cases will be insufficient to understand low-frequency adverse drug reactions such as drug-induced lung injuries in a clinical trial, and usually, this information is confirmed in a post-marketing survey. Although post-marketing all-case surveys have recently been conducted for many molecular-targeted drugs in Japan, drugs which had been developed before were investigated in ordinary post-marketing surveys or were self-reported data.

In considering ordinary post-marketing surveys compared to post-marketing all-case surveys, there is greater bias in the facility selection and there may be fewer occurrence rates of adverse drug reactions. Many facilities selected for post-marketing surveys for the field of cancer treatment are large with many cases and sufficient equipment. Thus, compared to the real world, the percentage of cases in good systemic conditions may become higher, and it must be kept in mind that the information of the prognosis after appearance of the events may come from facilities with sufficient intensive-care equipment.

Table 10.1 Incidence of lung injuries induced by anticancer drugs at the study step

Drug	Incidence	(n/N)
Irinotecan	1.3%	(11/847)
Vinorelbine	2.5%	(16/652)
Gemcitabine	1.5%	(5/329)
Amrubicin	2.2%	(4/181)
Paclitaxel	1.7%	(6/349)
Docetaxel	0%	(0/865)
Nedaplatin	0%	(0/530)
Nogitecan	0%	(0/530)

© The Author(s), under exclusive license to Springer Nature Singapore Pte Ltd. 2024
A. Gemma, *Analysis File of Drug-Induced Lung Injury*,
https://doi.org/10.1007/978-981-97-3446-7_10

10 Anticancer Drugs (TS-1, Taxanes, CPT-11, Platinum-Containing Drugs, Etc.)

10.1 Bleomycin (Bleo) (Fig. 10.1)

- Antitumor antibiotics.

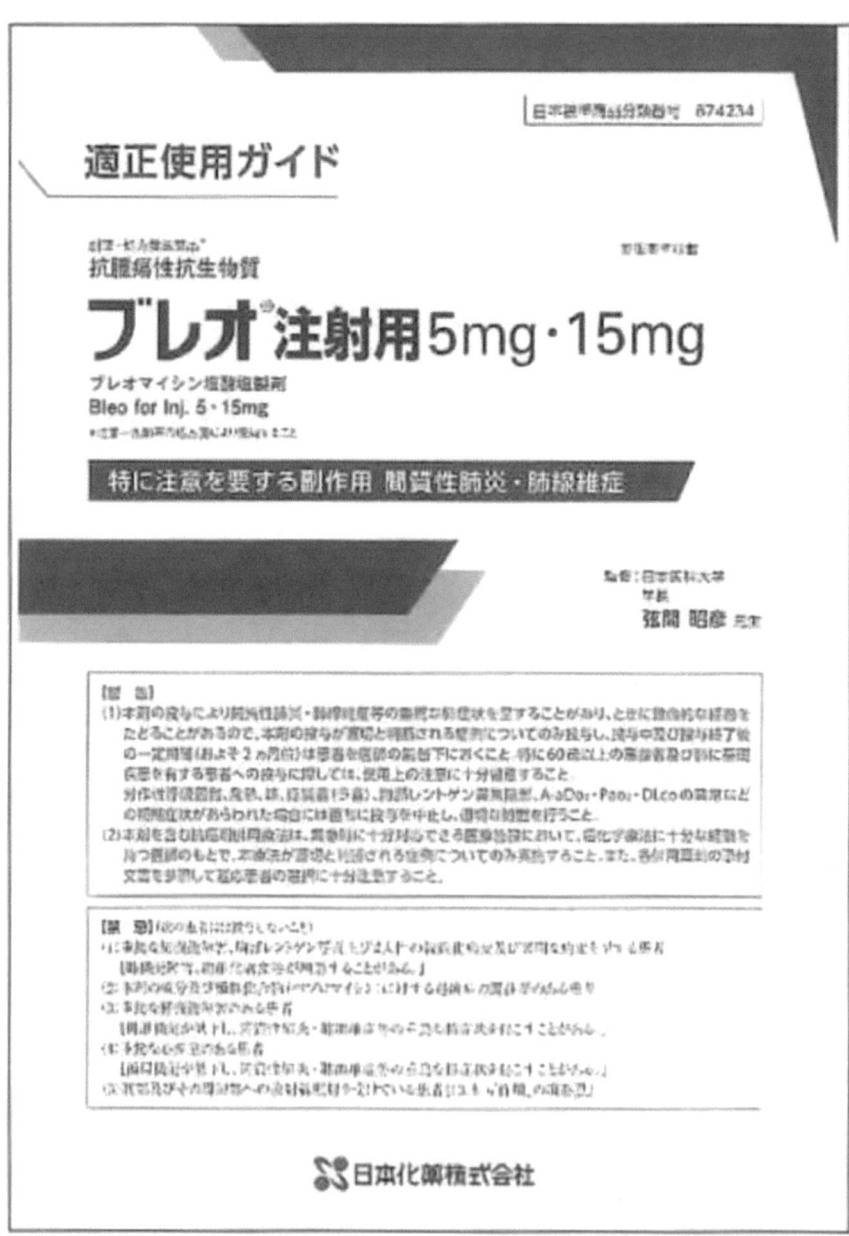

Fig. 10.1 Optimal clinical use guidelines of Bleo injection 5 mg and 15 mg. (Cited from Reference [1])

Fig. 10.2 Incidence in different total doses. (Created from Reference [1])

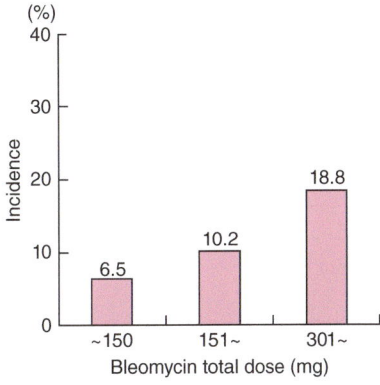

- Indications: (Injection) Skin cancer, head and neck cancer, lung cancer, esophagus cancer, malignant lymphoma, endocervical cancer, gliocytoma, thyroid cancer, germ cell tumor, (external use) skin malignant tumor.

Bleomycin is a known drug which induces drug-induced lung injury [2].

The incidence of drug-induced lung injuries was 10.2% [1]. The rate increased in accordance with increase in the total dose: 6.5% in 150 mg or less, 10.2% in 151–300 mg, and 18.8% in 301 mg or higher (Fig. 10.2).

10.1.1 Findings from the Surveys

The total dose and the incidence of drug-induced lung injuries are correlated, and the total recommended dose is 300 mg or less. Even in excessive cases caused by the combined therapy, the dose must be 360 mg or less. However, the relationship with the severity is not clear.

Incidence increases with older age, and the decrease in the dose must be considered when administered to patients aged 60 or older.

As the drug is basically eliminated by renal excretion, the evaluation of the renal function is important and the combination of radiation therapy and G-CSF may increase the risk of drug-induced lung injuries.

Administration is contraindicated in cases of apparent existing interstitial pneumonia detected by chest radiographs.

10.2 CPT-11 (Topotecin, Campto) (Fig. 10.3)

- Topoisomerase I inhibitor.
- Indications: Small cell lung cancer, non-small cell lung cancer, endocervical cancer, ovary cancer, gastric cancer (inoperable or recurrent), colon/rectal cancer

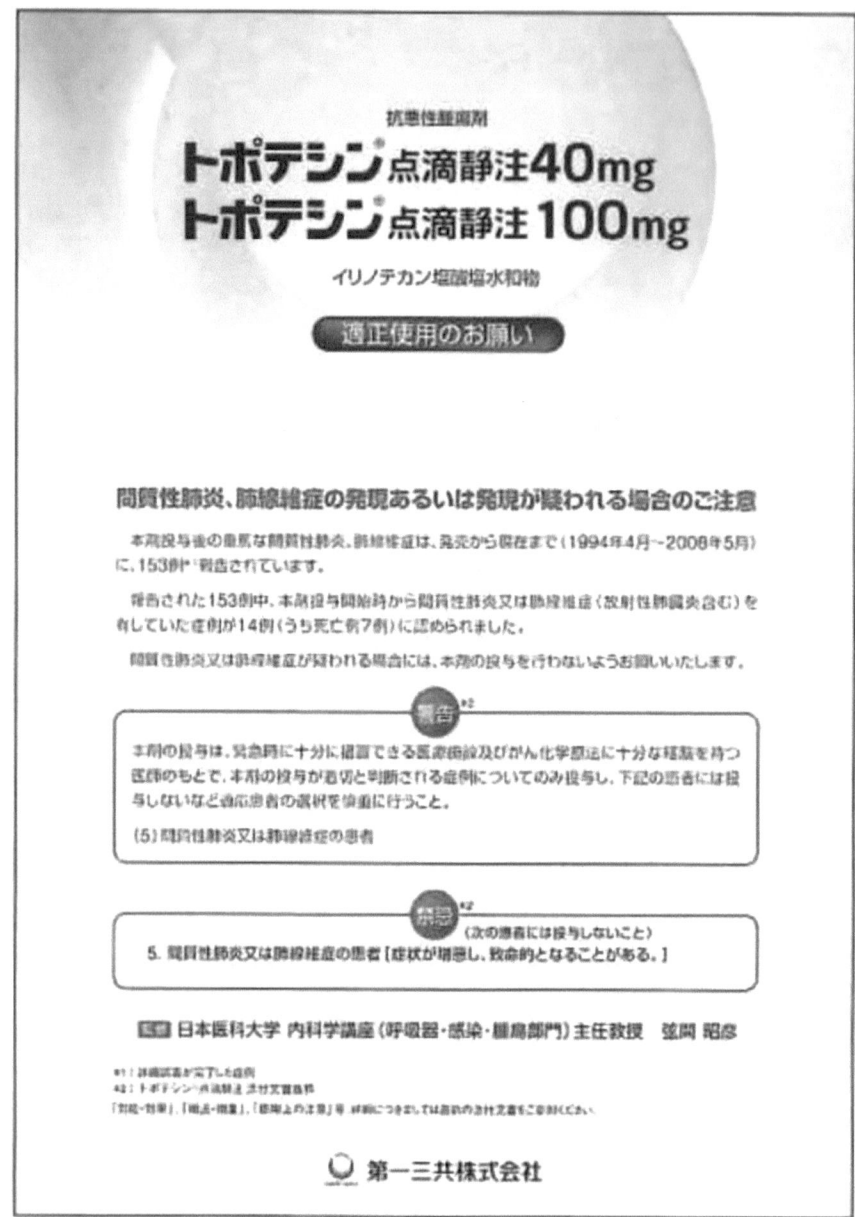

Fig. 10.3 Request for optimal use of Topotecin drip infusion. (Cited from Reference [3])

(inoperable or recurrent), breast cancer (inoperable or recurrent), spinocellular cancer, malignant lymphoma (non-Hodgkin's lymphoma), pediatric malignant solid tumor, and healing-unresectable pancreatic cancer.

10.2 CPT-11 (Topotecin, Campto)

There were 134 cases (0.9%) of interstitial pneumonia in 15,385 subjects followed in post-marketing surveys. The information is relatively old. Therefore, cautions about the appearance of interstitial pneumonia and pulmonary fibrosis have been added to the "Requests for optimal use of the drug" as a result of recent findings from the post-marketing study [3, 4].

10.2.1 Post-Marketing Appearance of Side Effects of Interstitial Lung Diseases

Topotecin [3].
　Subjects: Patients using Topotecin and reporting ILDs.
　Number of subjects: 153 cases.
　Study period: April 1994–May 2008.
　Results
37 deaths in which interstitial pneumonia may be involved. Among those cases, 14 subjects had interstitial pneumonia or pulmonary fibrosis at the start of administration, and 7 of those resulted in death.

Campto.
　Subjects: Patients using Campto and reporting ILDs.
　Number of subjects: 176 cases.
　Study period: April 1994–July 2006.
　Results
44 deaths in which interstitial pneumonia may be involved. Among those cases, 12 subjects had interstitial pneumonia or pulmonary fibrosis at the start of administration, and 4 of those resulted in death.

Analysis of image pattern (Topotecin) [1].
　Number of subjects: 18 cases whose disease type could be evaluated.
　Results
7 cases of HP pattern, 6 cases of DAD pattern, 3 cases of OP pattern, 1 case of HP + OP pattern, and 1 case of NSIP pattern.

10.2.2 Findings from the Surveys

If interstitial pneumonia appears, the prognosis is poor, particularly when there are existing lesions such as interstitial pneumonia. Surveys other than post-marketing all-case surveys show the appearance of drug-induced lung injuries in different cancer types (Fig. 10.4). Although the frequency is unknown because the parameter is

Fig. 10.4 Fatality rate in different cancer types. (Cited from Reference [4])

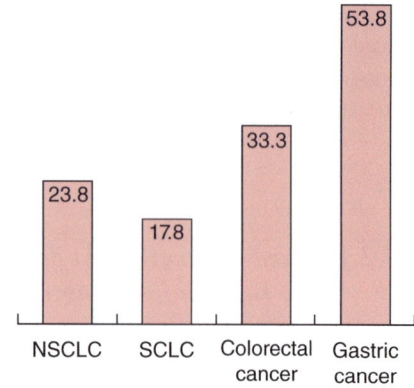

unknown, the prognosis may be different among the organs. With TS-1, the difference exists among primary organs, as explained the details in the item.

The image pattern was the typical pattern for drug-induced lung injuries.

In addition, in another paper about CT analysis, it was reported that serious ILD was found in 0.74% and the deaths in 0.17% [5] in 66 cases.

10.3 Tegafur/Gimeracil/Oteracil Potassium Combination Drugs (TS-1) (Fig. 10.5)

- Antipyrimidine.
- Indications: Gastric cancer, colon/rectal cancer, head and neck cancer, non-small cell lung cancer, inoperable or recurrent breast cancer, pancreas cancer, and biliary tract cancer.

10.3.1 Achievement Surveys for Lung Cancer/Other cancers [6]

Lung cancer.
 Study period: January 2005–December 2006.
 Subjects: Patients with non-small cell lung cancer.
 Number of subjects: Registered 1784 cases (collected 1708 cases and 1669 cases for safety evaluation).
 Observation period: Three courses (one course: 42 days [continuous administration for 28 days and drug holidays for 14 days]).
 Results: Reference [6].
 ILD incidence: 0.66% (11 cases).

10.3 Tegafur/Gimeracil/Oteracil Potassium Combination Drugs (TS-1)

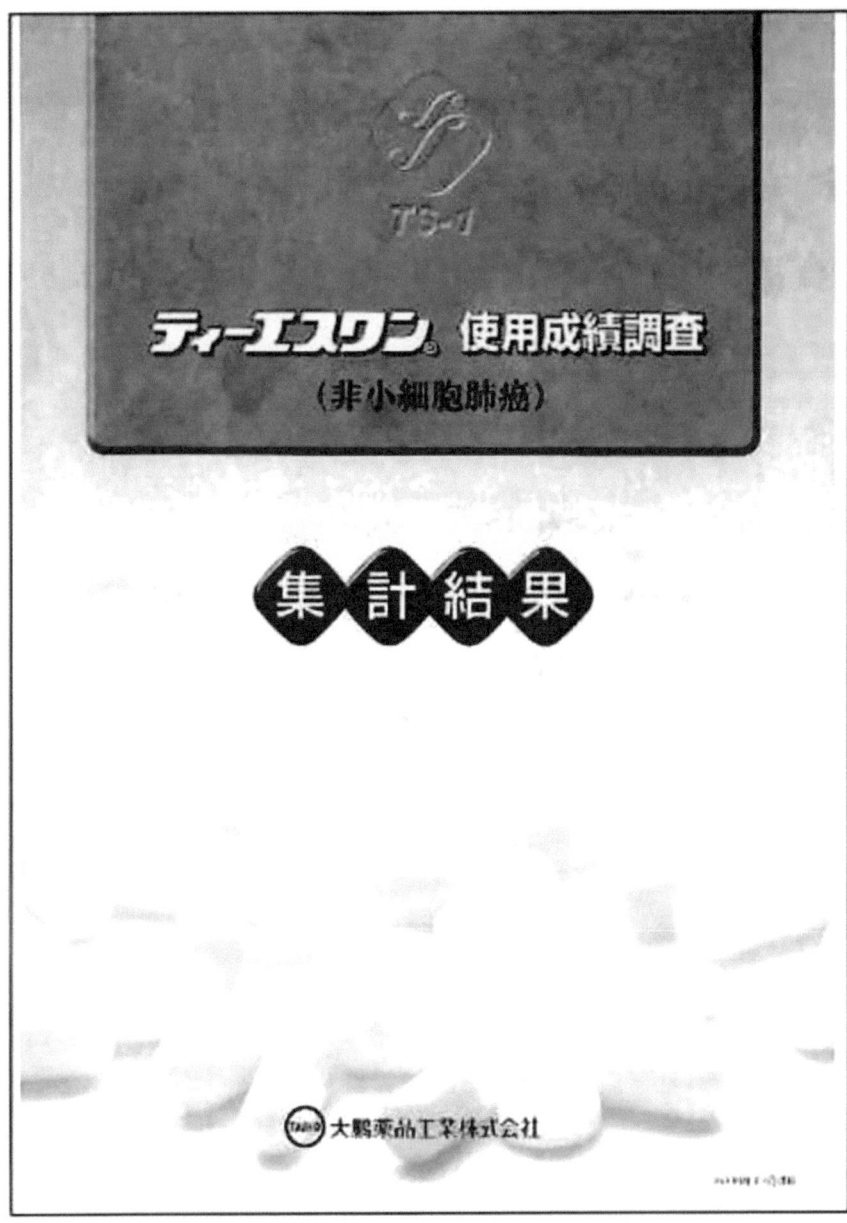

Fig. 10.5 Surveys for usage achievement of TS-1 (non-small cell lung cancer)

Table 10.2 Analysis of risk factors (logistic regression analysis)

Background factors	Variable		Odds ratio	95% CI
Allergic predisposition	Absence		1	1.057–16.322
	Presence		4.153	
Complications (interstitial pneumonia)	Absence		1	3.048–45.541
	Presence		11.782	
Medical history (interstitial pneumonia)	Absence		1	3.140–100.321
	Presence		17.749	
Combined antimalignant tumor drugs (other than CDDP)	Absence		1	1.085–11.055
	Presence		3.463	

Study factors: Sex, inpatient/outpatient division, age, PS, usage object, allergic predisposition, smoking history, complications, medical history, history of surgery, history of radiation therapy, history of treatment with antimalignant tumor drug, combined antimalignant tumor drugs, combined drugs, combined radiation therapy, and pre-administration renal dysfunction. (Cited from Reference [6])

Risk factors: Persons with allergic predisposition, cases complicated with interstitial pneumonia, medical history, and cases combined with anticancer drug treatment (Table 10.2).

Organs other than lung cancer [1].

ILD incidence: 0.05% (2 of 3808 cases) in patients with gastric cancer, 0.07% (1 of 1361 cases) in patients with breast cancer, and 0.24% (1 of 421 cases) in patients with pancreatic cancer.

TS-1 study.

ILD incidence: 0.27% (2 of 751 cases) in the whole study and 1.74% (2 of 115 cases) in patients with non-small cell lung cancer.

Image patterns.

Number of subjects: 25 cases obtained sufficient image information.

Results

10 cases of DAD pattern (40%), 5 cases (20%) of HP pattern, 3 cases (12%) of OP pattern, and 4 cases of non-typical pattern.

10.3.2 Findings from the Surveys

Topics

The disorders are different among the organs

- According to the achievement surveys in other organs, ILDs appeared in cancers in other organs less often than those in non-small cell lung cancer.

---

[1] No appearances were reported in 375 cases of head and neck cancer and 394 cases of biliary tract cancer.

- The risk factors listed in the achievement surveys in patients with lung cancer may be different than that in patients with cancers in other organs.
- Compared to other anticancer drugs used for wide range of cancer types such as CPT-11, ILD incidence and fatality rate in patients with lung cancer tend to be higher. Two reasons are assumed for that:
  - Many lung cancer patients are smokers, who are likely to have various complications and damaged lungs.
  - The frequency of chest CT is so high that the ILD may be detected easily in lung cancer.

From the image patterns, characteristics of ILD with TS-1 are summarized as follows:

- The DAD pattern is seen most frequently. However, similar to the anti-EGFR antibody, the influence of the high proportion of gastrointestinal cancers must be taken into consideration. Among those cases, there were 6 deaths, including 3 deaths with a DAD pattern, a high percentage. Conversely, among 10 cases of interstitial pneumonia with the DAD pattern, there were 3 deaths, a relatively low level.
- Among the image findings, 4 cases of conventional patterns showed centrilobular-type granular shadows and 2 cases were close to a hypersensitive pneumonitis induced by an inhalant antigen. The hypersensitive pneumonitis case may occur accidentally by inhaling the antigen.

For platinum-containing drugs, the package insert was revised to add considerations for drug-induced lung injuries when using oxaliplatin or miriplatin hydrate.

10.4 Platinum-Containing Drugs: Oxaliplatin (Elplat)

- CDDP derivative, strong neural toxicity.
- Indications: Healing-unresectable advanced/recurrent colon/rectal cancer, adjunctive chemotherapy after colon cancer surgery, healing-unresectable pancreatic cancer, gastric cancer, small intestinal cancer.

10.4.1 Achievement Surveys for the Usage [7]

Study period: 2005–2008 [7].
Subjects: Marketing surveys and self-reports.
Number of subjects: 4998 cases.
Results

ILD incidence: 0.26% (13 cases) (statistic results including self-reports: 118 cases of ILD and 46 fatal cases (39.0%) among the ILD cases).

Cases of pre-existing lung lesion at the start of the administration: 45 cases of lung metastasis, 12 cases of interstitial pneumonia/pulmonary fibrosis, and 10 cases of emphysema.

The fatality rate in interstitial pneumonia/pulmonary fibrosis cases was 66.7% (8 cases), which was higher than those without pre-existing lung lesions. However, it was not significant because of the insufficient number of the cases.

Analysis of image patterns.

Number of subjects: 26 image-evaluable cases including self-reports.

Results: (Table 10.3).

10 cases of DAD cases (38.5%), 7 cases of OP pattern (26.9%), 5 cases of HP pattern + OP pattern (15.4%), and 2 cases of HP pattern (7.7%).

Pre-existing lung diseases were detected in 11 of 26 cases, including 5 fatal cases [7].

Findings from the Surveys

FOLFOX4 or FOLFOX6 as a combined drug was administered to most of the subjects in the surveys. Basically, oxaliplatin is administered in patients with gastrointestinal diseases, and the cases are thus influenced by combined drugs. Accordingly, the analysis of causative drug in this event is so difficult that the combined therapy must be considered as a unit.

As for drug-induced lung injuries, although the fatality rate is high, originally, the incidence was low and it is thus unlikely to influence the treatment plan. At the step when the treatment is progressing, the balance with the effect must be re-considered.

Table 10.3 Disease-type patterns in 26 cases with administration of oxaliplatin

	Deaths	Cases other than deaths	Total
Diffuse alveolar damage (DAD) pattern	7[a]	3	10 (38.5%)
Organizing pneumonia (OP) pattern	2[b]	5	7 (26.9%)
Hypersensitive reaction (HR) + OP pattern	0	4	4 (15.4%)
HR pattern	0	2	2 (7.7%)
Unevaluable	1	2	3 (11.5%)
Total	10	16	26 (100.0%)

[a] In 1 of the 7 cases, this drug was administered continuously after the appearance of interstitial pneumonia on the images

[b] In both cases, the drug was administered continuously after the appearance of interstitial pneumonia on the images. (Cited from Reference [7])

10.5 Platinum-Containing Drugs: Miriplatin (Miripla)

- Indications: Lipiodolization in hepatic cell cancer.

Miriplatin is used with arteriography. Many subjects received the administration once. Reports on interstitial pneumonia after the launch of miriplatin were aggregated and were investigated by the evaluation committee of a third party.

10.5.1 Investigation by the Evaluation Committee of a Third Party

Study period: January 20, 2010–September 2012.
Subjects: ILD cases in about 26,000 estimated patients.
Number of subjects: 15 cases.
Results
Appearance of drug-induced interstitial pneumonia: 9 cases.
Fatal cases: 7 cases.
Onset time: Many cases within 1 week after administration.
Risk factors: Unknown.

10.5.2 Findings from the Surveys

Because of an insufficient number of the cases, factors such as risk factors could not be analyzed. The event appeared within 1 week in many cases.

Oxaliplatin is administered for a long period, whereas miriplatin is administered once. The onset time of interstitial pneumonia is inferred to result from the administration method rather than the features of the drug.

In 9 of 15 cases of ILD, the causal relationship with miriplatin is assumed not to be deniable. The fatality rate is high, in 7 of 15 cases [8].

10.6 Pemetrexed (Alimta)

- Multiple folate-metabolizing enzymes are inhibited at the same time and DNA synthesis is inhibited.
- Indications: Malignant pleural mesothelioma and unresectable advanced/recurrent non-small cell lung cancer.

Achievement surveys for specific usage in lung cancer (i) [9].
Study period: June 2009–May 2010.
Subjects: Patients with unresectable advanced/recurrent non-small cell lung cancer.
Number of subjects: 683 cases.
Observation period: 12 months.
Results
Incidence: 2.6% (18 cases), presence of existing ILD in 5 of 18 cases and 1.8% (12 cases) for severe ILD.
Achievement surveys for specific usage for patients with mesothelioma (ii) [10].
Subjects: Patients with malignant pleural mesothelioma.
Number of subjects: 903 cases.
Observation period: 12 months.
Results
Incidence: 1.6% (14 cases).
Cases of existing interstitial pneumonia: 7 cases.
Exacerbation cases: 3 of 7 cases.

10.6.1   Findings from the Surveys

The number is never small.

Risk factors listed are male, 60 years old or older, existing interstitial pneumonia, asbestosis with mesothelioma, and smoking with lung cancer.

The events are found in many subjects who had asbestos inhalation or smokers, in which the lung has been damaged. Thus, caution must be exercised.

In surveys of mesothelioma, existing interstitial pneumonia was found in 7 of 903 cases and exacerbation was found in 3 of the 7 cases, which is a high frequency.

10.7   Amrubicin (Calsed)

- Topoisomerase II inhibitor.
- Indications: Non-small cell lung cancer, small cell lung cancer.

10.8   Gemcitabine (Gemzar)

- Antipyrimidine.
- Indications: Non-small cell lung cancer, pancreatic cancer, biliary tract cancer, urothelial cancer, inoperative or recurrent breast cancer, ovarian cancer worsened after cancer chemotherapy, recurrent/refractory malignant lymphoma.

10.8.1 Single-Facility Consecutive Surveys

Amrubicin (Report on Japanese Cases) [11, 12].
  ILD incidence: 7% (7/100 cases), 3.3% (3/92 cases).
Gemcitabine[13].
  Number of subjects: 890 cases (855 cases for the safety analysis).
  Results
  ILD incidence: 0.7% (6 cases).

10.8.2 Findings from the Surveys

Gemcitabine-induced lung injuries are known to be found with mild ground glass-like shadows in many cases, and an incidence of 7–8% (9 of 118 cases) is reported [14].

For amrubicin and gemcitabine, in case that apparent interstitial pneumonia (pulmonary fibrosis) is an existing lesion, administration is prohibited in Japan.

Compared to CPT-11 (which is prohibited in cases of existing interstitial pneumonia [pulmonary fibrosis]), it is important to note that cases with low risks are selected by the doctors of lung cancer specialist.

References

1. Optimal clinical use guidelines of Bleo injection 5 mg and 15 mg. Nippon Kayaku Co., Ltd. 2020.
2. Rossi SE, et al. Radiographics. 2000;20:1245–59.
3. Topotecin injection, irinotecan hydrochloride: CPT-11. Daiichi Sankyo Co., Ltd. Revised in June 2008.
4. Requests for optimal use of Campto injection (irinotecan hydrochloride: CPT-11). Cautions in case of appearance of interstitial pneumonia or pulmonary fibrosis and in suspected cases. Yakult Honsha Co., Ltd.
5. Yoshii N, et al. Anti-Cancer Drugs. 2011;22:563–8.
6. Ito K. Gan To Kagaku Ryoho. 2015;42:595–603.
7. Requests for usage of Elplat injection 50 mg and 100 mg and Elplat drip infusion 50 mg and 100 mg. Yakult Honsha Co., Ltd. 2010.
8. Appearance of interstitial pneumonia with Miripla injection 70 mg, Miripla suspension 4 mL. Sumitomo Dainippon Pharma Co., Ltd. Revised in December 2019.
9. Report on the final analysis results of specific surveys for usage achievement of Alimta® (non-small cell lung cancer). Eli Lilly Japan K.K. 2009.
10. Anon. Report on the final analysis results of specific surveys (all-case surveys) for usage achievement of Alimta® (malignant pleural mesothelioma). Chuo-ku Kobe: Eli Lilly Japan K.K.; 2013.
11. Yoh K, Kenmotsu H, Yamaguchi Y, et al. J Thorac Oncol. 2010;5:1435–8.
12. Miura Y, Saito Y, Atsumi K, et al. Jpn J Clin Oncol. 2016;46:674–80.
13. Ioka T, Katayama K, Tanaka S, et al. Jpn J Clin Oncol. 2013;43:139–45.
14. Umemura S, Yamane H, Suwaki T, et al. Cancer Res Clin Oncol. 2011;137:1469–75.

Index

A
Afatinib, 8, 15, 17–21, 28–29
Afinitor, 47–57
Alecensa, 82
Alectinib, 79–82, 84–86, 89
Alimta, 111–112
Amrubicin, 101, 112, 113
Antibody-drug conjugate (ADC), 91, 94–98
Anti-cancer drug, 6, 7, 11, 15, 44, 47, 56, 74, 101–103, 105–113
Anti-EGFR antibody, 39, 109
Atezolizumab, 9, 63–74
Avastin, 77

B
Bevacizumab, 75–77
Bleo, 102–103
Bleomycin, 3, 44, 102–103
Bortezomib, 10, 59–62

C
Calsed, 112
Campto, 103–106
Caprelsa, 34
Cetuximab, 37–40, 42–45
CPT-11, 44, 101–113
Crizotinib, 8, 79–82, 85–86, 89

D
Durvalumab, 63–74

E
EGFR inhibitors, 15, 17–21, 80
Elplat, 109–110
Emtansine, 91, 95–98
Enhertu, 94–98
Erbitux, 37–41
Erlotinib, 8, 10, 11, 15, 17–29
Everolimus, 47–57

G
Gefitinib, 6, 7, 15, 17–22, 24, 28, 29
Gemcitabine, 24, 27, 45, 101, 112–113
Gemzar, 112–113
Gilotrif, 28–29

H
Herceptin, 85–86

I
Ibrance, 89–90
Imfinzi, 72–74
Immune checkpoint inhibitor(s), 8–9, 31, 33, 63–74
Iressa, 6, 15–21, 80

K
Kadcyla, 91–94
Keytruda, 69–72

M
Miripla/Miriplatin, 109, 111
mTOR inhibitor(s), 4–6, 8–9, 47, 48, 50–53, 55, 56

N
Necitumumab, 37, 39, 40, 42–45
Neoangiogenesis inhibitors, 75–77
Nexavar, 10, 76–77
Nivolumab, 9, 10, 31–33, 44, 63–74

O
Opdivo, 63–69
Osimertinib, 15, 17–21, 29–34, 74
Oxaliplatin, 109–111

P
Palbociclib, 89–90
Panitumumab, 37, 39, 40, 42–45
Pembrolizumab, 9, 63–74
Pemetrexed, 111–112
Perjeta, 86–89
Personal genetic predisposition, 6
Pertuzumab, 86–89
Platinum-containing drug, 95, 101–103, 105–113
Portrazza, 45
Proteasome inhibitor, 59, 60, 62

S
Sorafenib, 10, 75–77
Sunitinib, 75–77
Sutent, 75–76

T
Tagrisso, 29–34
Tarceva, 22–28, 80
T-DM1, 91–95
Tecentriq, 72
Tegafur/gimeracil/oteracil potassium combination drug, 106–109
Temsirolimus, 47, 48, 50–56
Topotecin, 103–106
Torisel, 47
Trastuzumab, 85–86, 91, 94–98
Trastuzumab deruxtecan, 94–98
Trastuzumab emtansine, 91–94
TS-1, 10, 44, 101–103, 105–113

V
Vandetanib, 34
Vectibix, 42–45
Velcade, 59–62

X
Xalkori, 79–81

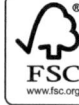

MIX
Papier aus verantwortungsvollen Quellen
Paper from responsible sources
FSC® C105338

If you have any concerns about our products,
you can contact us on
ProductSafety@springernature.com

In case Publisher is established outside the EU,
the EU authorized representative is:
Springer Nature Customer Service Center GmbH
Europaplatz 3, 69115 Heidelberg, Germany

Printed by Libri Plureos GmbH
in Hamburg, Germany